ABG INTERPRETATION:

Everything You Need To Know To

Interpret Arterial Blood Gases

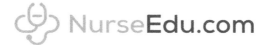

Disclaimer:

Although the author and publisher have made every effort to ensure that the information in this book was correct at press time, the author and publisher do not assume and hereby disclaim any liability to any party for any loss, damage, or disruption caused by errors or omissions, whether such errors or omissions result from negligence, accident, or any other cause.

This book is not intended as a substitute for the medical advice of physicians. The reader should regularly consult a physician in matters relating to his/her health and particularly with respect to any symptoms that may require diagnosis or medical attention.

NCLEX®, NCLEX®-RN, and NCLEX®-PN are registered trademarks of the National Council of State Boards of Nursing, Inc. They hold no affiliation with this product.

Some images within this book are either royalty-free images, used under license from their respective copyright holders, or images that are in the public domain.

ISBN: 978-1-952914-00-3

FREE BONUS

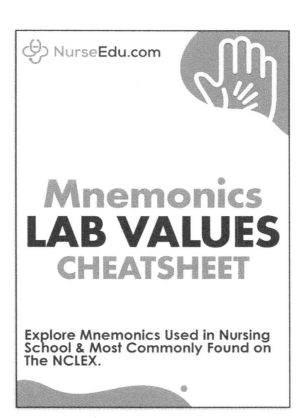

FREE Download – Just Visit:

NurseEdu.com/bonus

Table of Contents

Table of Contents

Chapter One:

INTRODUCTION

The arterial blood gases (or ABGs) are some of the more difficult lab tests to understand in all of medicine. Sure, there are normal results given along with the test values, but it doesn't end there. What does a certain pH in the blood mean? Where does the bicarbonate level come from? These components, along with other values, need to be understood so you can interpret them.

Basically, the ABGs are a test of the arterial blood that check the oxygen levels, the carbon dioxide levels, the acidity (or pH) of the blood, the oxyhemoglobin saturation, and the bicarbonate. If you have a fancy blood gas analyzer, you can get a methemoglobin level, a carboxyhemoglobin level, and sometimes just a hemoglobin level. Each of these lab tests reveal crucial values that are important in caring for patients in the intensive care unit (ICU) and other hospital settings. If you do not know what oxyhemoglobin saturation means (or any of these values), never fear! By the time you finish this guide, you will be an old pro.

What is an ABG?

An ABG (or "blood gas") is a group of tests that are not only drawn together, they are interpreted together, and they have special meaning when they are interpreted. It is important to remember that true "blood gases" are checked on arterial blood, meaning the sample must be taken out of an artery. We will talk about venous blood gases too, but these do not provide the same information as arterial blood gas. Unless we say otherwise, blood gases should be recognized as being of arterial origin.

The blood gases are important because they say a lot about the metabolic processes going on inside the body. Is there a metabolic disorder, where too much acid is being made by the body? Is there a respiratory problem, which can affect oxygenation and acid-base levels in the body? Could there be kidney disease that does not allow the kidneys to regulate the acids and bases inside the body?

You need to know that the main goal of acid-base function in the body is to keep the pH of the bloodstream as normal as possible. A normal blood pH is between 7.35 and 7.45. Blood that has a lower pH than this is called "acidotic," meaning it has "acidosis"—a large amount of acid in the body. Blood that has a higher pH is "alkalinic," meaning it has "alkalosis." In other words, there are too many bases in the body.

The body normally produces acids as part of normal metabolic processes and CO2 (carbon dioxide) is one of them, even though it is a gas and is itself not an acid. (Consider CO2 as an acid for all practical purposes here.) Another acid that is made by the body is lactic acid, which is made by muscles that engage in an aerobic activity. These acids must be regulated through the body's acid-base mechanisms and the ABGs give you a window to see into these processes.

The lungs exhale CO2, which is one mechanism that regulates the acids in the body. The kidneys will excrete or conserve hydrogen ions (acids) or hydroxyl ions (bases) in order to keep the body's pH as normal as possible. The lungs and kidneys can increase or decrease their ability to do this in order to compensate for acidosis or alkalosis. In addition, the lungs bring in oxygen, which is measured by the ABG.

The acid-base balance is crucial to the pH of the blood. The pH of the blood is important because enzymes in the body depend on a specific pH range. If the pH becomes too abnormal, the body will suffer the effects.

There are many acute and chronic processes that can affect the ABGs. Kidney problems can impact the pH balance and problems with lung function can affect both oxygenation and the acid-base metabolism. Other diseases that can affect the blood pH include uncontrolled diabetes (which can cause ketoacidosis and acid buildup in the body), anxiety, shock, prolonged vomiting, or severe diarrhea, to name a few.

The ABGs give a brief snapshot as to what is going on with the patient's arterial blood. It measures the following:

- Arterial pH—this is a measure of the acidity or alkalinity of the blood. Increased acids or CO_2 in the bloodstream will decrease the pH, while increased bicarbonate or decreased CO_2 will increase the pH.
- Partial pressure of oxygen, or PaO_2—this is a measurement of the amount of arterial oxygen in the bloodstream.
- Partial pressure of CO_2, or $PaCO_2$—this measures the amount of carbon dioxide in the arterial bloodstream. As the $PaCO_2$ goes up, the pH decreases so the blood becomes acidic. As the $PaCO_2$ goes down, the pH goes up, making the arterial blood more basic or alkaline.
- Oxygen saturation—this is referred to as the O_2Sat or SaO_2 level. It is the percent of the blood's hemoglobin that is currently carrying oxygen. Most of the hemoglobin will be oxygenated, so this oxygen saturation level will be high (greater than 95 percent). Oxygen saturation can also be obtained through a pulse oximetry reading.
- Oxygen content—this is described as the CaO_2 or O_2CT. It is the amount of oxygen contained in 100 milliliters of blood.
- Bicarbonate, or HCO_3- level—this is the main way that CO_2 is carried in the bloodstream. It is released and reabsorbed by the kidneys in response to imbalances in

4

the blood pH level. Bicarbonate is a basic or alkaline substance so, as the level goes up, the pH level increases. Your blood will also carry bicarbonate to the lungs for it to be exhaled as carbon dioxide.

- Base excess or base deficit—this indicates the amount of excess or insufficient levels of bicarbonate in the blood. If there is a negative base excess, then there is an increased level of acid in the blood. It is an important factor to consider when deciding how to correct the pH imbalance of the patient's blood.

ABG versus VBG: What is the Difference?

The arterial blood gases are unique because they are done on arterial blood, where the oxygen content should be the highest. It gives a good representation of the gases contained within the bloodstream. Venous blood gases, on the other hand, are done on venous blood draws. The venous blood can give a good idea of the CO_2 level, bicarbonate level, and pH of the blood but cannot accurately indicate the oxygenation of the blood. Only arterial blood gases can accurately do this.

The biggest problem with arterial blood gases is that they are difficult to obtain. Try it sometime on a patient that is unconscious who needs an ABG done and you will see how hard it is. Why an unconscious patient? This is because getting arterial blood gases is extremely painful. If the patient has a weak pulse or if this is your first time, it will be all that much harder.

This makes venous blood gases a more attractive option and retrieving them can be performed without much difficulty. There are still other ways to assess ventilation, blood pH, and oxygenation besides the arterial blood gases and these will be covered in this chapter.

Venous blood gases or VBGs can be obtained from a peripheral venous sample, a mixed venous sample (from a pulmonary artery catheter), or a central venous sample (from a central venous catheter). A central venous sample is preferred if the patient has central venous access already. Do not place a pulmonary artery catheter or central venous catheter just to get VBGs. Use them only if they are available to you. Do not obtain a peripheral venous sample with a tourniquet on because the ischemia below the tourniquet level will obscure the results.

The VBG will measure the oxygen tension in the veins, the carbon dioxide tension in the veins, the venous pH, the bicarbonate level, and the venous oxyhemoglobin saturation. The most valuable parts of this evaluation are the $PvCO_2$, the pH, and the bicarbonate level. These results can help to assess the patient's acid-base status. In addition, the SvO_2 (percent saturation of oxygen in the venous hemoglobin) can help direct therapy in cases of septic shock or severe septicemia. The partial pressure of oxygen in the veins or PvO_2 does not have a real practical value.

The $PaCO_2$, pH, and bicarbonate levels will roughly correlate with the arterial blood levels with some small differences. The central venous pH will be 0.03 to 0.05 units lower than the arterial pH. The PCO_2 will be 4 to 5 mm Hg greater, but the bicarbonate should be the same. In peripheral venous blood the PCO_2 will be 3 to 8 mm Hg higher than in the arterial blood, and the bicarbonate will be 1 to 2 mEq/L higher. The peripheral pH will be 0.03 to 0.04 units lower than in the arterial blood. You should always periodically compare the venous and arterial blood gases in your patient.

You can also measure the end-tidal CO_2 level or $PetCO_2$ level in your patient, which is noninvasive and can estimate the arterial carbon dioxide level. This test is also called capnography. The patient wears a tightly fitted mask and a sample of the expired gas is obtained. The amount of CO_2 in expired air is within a mm Hg of the $PaCO_2$, but only in relatively healthy people. It is a less accurate test in the ICU, where patients are sicker. It is also used to a greater degree in the NICU and in operating rooms to evaluate ventilation.

There are systems that measure transcutaneous CO_2 levels, which is like pulse oximetry. Pulse oximetry measures the $ptcCO_2$ level. The test must be done after warming the skin to 42-45 degrees Celsius. It then requires an electrode that is placed on the patient's skin to measure transcutaneous CO_2 levels. This test is more accurate in neonates than it is on a sick adult with poor perfusion, and it is less accurate when the

PaCO2 level is greater than 56 mm Hg. Still, this is a noninvasive test that does have some applications in critical care medicine. Abnormal test results should be confirmed with an ABG test.

What do the ABGs tell me besides what we've already talked about?

The main goal of the arterial blood gas is to obtain and interpret the pH, PaCO2, bicarbonate, PaO2, and oxygen saturation levels. But there is no need to do another venous sampling if you need to have electrolytes, hemoglobin, or hematocrit levels drawn. The arterial blood gas blood can check these levels accurately as well.

When are ABGs used in the clinical setting?

Arterial blood gases can be checked for many different reasons. Think about doing ABGs in the following situations:

- Kidney failure
- Uncontrolled diabetes
- Shock
- Trauma
- Lung failure
- COPD/Asthma
- Hemorrhage
- Chemical poisoning

- Metabolic disease
- Drug overdose

Anytime you think there might be an acid-base disturbance, you should consider obtaining an ABG to further evaluate your patient. If you are treating a patient with respiratory failure or diabetic ketoacidosis, you will need the ABG to evaluate the patient's progress. In certain situations, you will want to know the patient's carboxyhemoglobin level or the methemoglobin level and the ABG is how you can access this information. In rare situations, such as in severe trauma or hypotension, an arterial sampling may be all you can get.

Contraindications for obtaining an ABG include an abnormal modified Allen's test (more on that later), infection or thrombus at the puncture site, severe peripheral vascular disease, and Raynaud's syndrome. Sometimes, you can get an alternative site. Some relative contraindications include being on thrombolytic therapy, having a coagulopathy, or a low platelet count. People with mild bleeding problems may be able to have a needle stick but not an indwelling arterial catheter.

Why do we need to know ABGs?

The arterial blood gas is a unique test that does not, of course, need to be performed on many patients. Sick ICU patients with possible acidemia or respiratory failure can only really be adequately managed by monitoring their ABGs. This is the only real way to obtain the acid-base data necessary to treat a very sick patient. Pulse oximeters have largely replaced performing an arterial blood gas on a possibly hypoxic patient. Sometimes the pulse oximetry reading can be inaccurate or impossible to obtain, however, which makes an arterial blood gas measurement necessary.

CHAPTER QUESTIONS

1. Which aspect of the arterial blood gas analysis can be obtained through other means besides the ABGs?

    a. PaO2
    b. PaCO2
    c. SaO2
    d. CaO2

Answer: **c.** The SaO2 (or percent oxygen saturation) can be obtained through a pulse oximetry analysis and, in most cases, these two results will be equivalent.

2. Which measurement on an arterial blood gas analysis measures the degree of acidity or alkalinity of the arterial blood?

    a. pH
    b. PaCO2
    c. PaO2
    d. HCO3-

Answer: **a.** The pH of the blood is a direct measurement of the acidity or alkalinity of arterial blood.

3. Which measurement on an arterial blood gas analysis is mainly a measure of the bases in the bloodstream?

    a. pH
    b. PaCO2
    c. PaO2
    d. HCO3-

Answer: **d.** The HCO3- level, or bicarbonate level, is mainly a measure of the bases in the bloodstream. Bicarbonate is a basic substance.

4. Which pH level would be indicative of arterial blood that is acidotic?

    a. 7.25
    b. 7.35
    c. 7.45
    d. 7.55

Answer: **a.** Acidosis of the arterial blood means that the pH is too low. A normal pH level is 7.35 to 7.45, so an arterial pH that is below this level would be considered acidotic.

5. Which value will be least similar in comparing an arterial blood gas and a venous blood gas sample?

    a. HCO3-
    b. PaCO2
    c. PaO2
    d. pH

Answer: **c.** The PaO2, or the partial pressure of oxygen, will be very different when comparing arterial blood and venous blood because oxygen gets consumed in the tissues, before the venous oxygen level is drawn. This makes the oxygen value less in venous blood compared to arterial blood.

6. What is measured in a capnography test?

    a. Partial pressure of oxygen
    b. Fraction of inspired air that is oxygen
    c. Bicarbonate level in arterial blood
    d. End-tidal carbon dioxide level

Answer: **d.** Capnography evaluates the amount of carbon dioxide in the expired air, so it measures the end-tidal carbon dioxide level, which can help evaluate the partial pressure of carbon dioxide in the patient.

7. What will the difference in the central venous blood pH be in comparison to the arterial blood pH?

    a. 1-2 units higher
    b. The same as arterial blood
    c. 0.03 to 0.05 units lower
    d. 0.5-0.7 units lower

Answer: **c.** The central venous blood pH will be close to that measured in arterial blood, but it will be 0.03 to 0.05 units lower than arterial blood.

8. What value will usually be the same when measuring central venous blood and arterial blood?

    a. Bicarbonate
    b. Partial pressure of oxygen
    c. pH
    d. Partial pressure of carbon dioxide

Answer: **a.** When comparing central venous blood and arterial blood, only the bicarbonate level will be the same in both samples.

Chapter Two:

A BIT OF ABG SCIENCE

We have thrown around some big terms, like oxygen tension and partial pressure of carbon dioxide, without really explaining what they mean. In order to really understand what it all means, we must go back and talk about gases in solutions, gases in other gases, and what happens to oxygen and carbon dioxide in the blood.

Partial Pressure of Gases

In the real world, gases are rarely seen in their purest form. Even air is a mixture of gases, and the gases inside the bloodstream form as mixtures as well. This leads to the idea of partial pressures. The "total" pressure of a mixture of gases is the pressure a gas would exert on the walls of a closed vessel.

In the atmosphere, there is not any kind of a vessel, but there is a pressure called the "atmospheric pressure" that exists at the surface of the earth. At sea level, the weight of pressure on things like the ground and people are set at one atmosphere, or about 760 mm Hg (which stands for millimeters of mercury). As you go to higher elevations, the atmospheric pressure is less, which is why it is harder to breathe at extremely high elevations.

In the air, there is nitrogen (the most prevalent gas), oxygen, water vapor, and carbon dioxide (the least prevalent gas). Each of these gases exerts a separate pressure that adds up to the total pressure of air. This leads to Dalton's law of partial pressures, which states that the sum of the partial pressures of all gases in a mixture equals the total pressure.

Typical dry air is about 78 percent nitrogen gas and about 21 percent oxygen gas with very little water vapor and carbon dioxide. If the total pressure of the atmosphere is 760 millimeters of mercury, the partial pressure of nitrogen is 78 percent of that, or about 600 mm Hg, and the partial pressure of oxygen is 21 percent of that, or about 160 mm Hg. **Figure 1 shows what this looks like:**

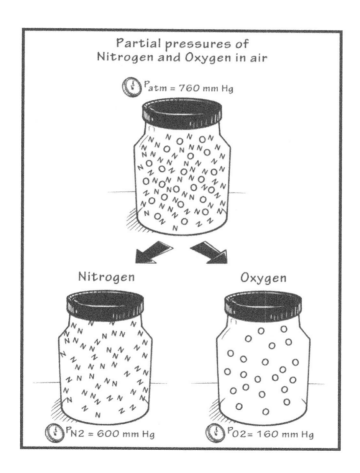

In the bloodstream, gases can dissolve just as they can

dissolve in any liquid. Not all gases dissolve to the same degree though. Nitrogen, for example, does not dissolve well in liquid blood, so you do not usually have to deal with that. Carbon dioxide dissolves in liquids, which is why it is seen in a can of soda. These types of gas molecules dissolve like salt dissolves in a solution. They dissolve to an equilibrium state so that the partial pressure of the gas in the liquid is the same as the partial pressure of the gas in the surrounding air.

There are other forms of gas in the blood that do not contribute to this equilibrium between the liquid (dissolved) state and the gaseous state. Gases that are bound to proteins (such as hemoglobin and oxygen) do not contribute to the partial pressure of the gas in a solution. This is how a lot of oxygen can get from place to place in the blood.

Gases that become chemically modified also do not contribute to the partial pressure of the gas. Carbon dioxide will sometimes convert to carbonic acid in the blood, which is not a gas. There is also an equilibrium state between CO_2 gas and bicarbonate. Bicarbonate is also not a gas, so it does not contribute to the partial pressure of CO_2 in the bloodstream.

This leads us to Henry's Law. Henry's law states that the concentration of the gas in a liquid depends on the partial pressure of the gas in the liquid, as well as on the unique chemical properties of the liquid and the gas. The unique chemical properties lead to a "gas constant" that depends on the nature of the gas and liquid. It states that the concentration of the gas = (constant) x (partial pressure of the gas in the liquid). **Figure 2 describes this phenomenon:**

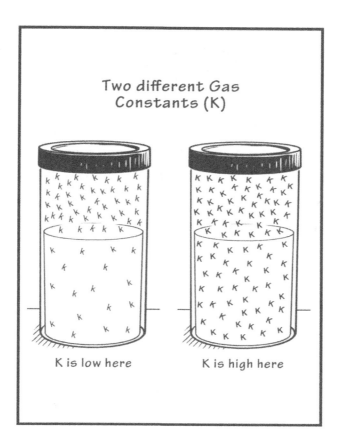

Two different Gas
Constants (K)

K is low here   K is high here

Gas Exchange in the Lungs

Oxygen and carbon dioxide must get across an alveolar membrane in order to get from the liquid (dissolved) state to the gaseous state. This is a lot easier than you would think. It is not an active transport process; it happens through the diffusion of gases across the membrane, which is very thin.

Fick's Law determines the rate at which gases cross the alveolar membrane.

According to Fick's law, the rate of diffusion of a gas across a membrane depends on the membrane itself, the surface area of the membrane, the thickness of the membrane, and the partial pressure gradient of the gas across the permeable membrane. The rate of diffusion depends on a specific diffusion coefficient for the gas and the membrane together, the surface area, the partial pressure difference, and divided by the membrane thickness. **Figure 3 shows Fick's law, in which V'gas is the rate of gas diffusion:**

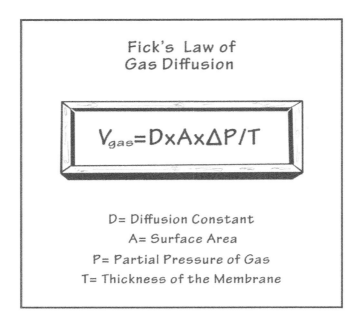

Gases diffuse more easily across the alveolar membrane because the membrane is thin and has a very large surface area. There will be differences in the partial pressures of the gases that will determine how fast it crosses the membrane.

The exact diffusing capacity of oxygen and carbon dioxide is difficult to determine because the partial pressure of these gases change as the gases travel through the pulmonary capillaries. Therefore, doctors measure the DLCO, or diffusing capacity of carbon monoxide, when determining if gases are passing through the alveoli. CO gas binds tightly to hemoglobin and it has nearly zero partial pressure in the pulmonary capillaries (because all of it is bound). Measuring the amount that can diffuse across the membrane is a good way to evaluate the membrane itself and to determine how well oxygen and carbon dioxide pass through the membrane.

Some gases have diffusion-limited gas exchange, meaning the actual diffusion depends on how fast it can get across the membrane as blood flows through it. This is true of carbon monoxide and that's why it is used to check for lung damage to the alveoli.

Other gases have perfusion-limited gas exchange. This means that the gas travels fast across the membrane and is limited by the rate of blood flow through the capillaries. An example of this is nitrous oxide, which is not changed at all as it passes through the gas to liquid phase. Blood values rise quickly, even if the alveolar membrane is not very effective at passing gas through it. The flow of blood, rather than the membrane itself, determines how much gets into the liquid.

So, what about oxygen? It turns out that oxygen diffuses rather quickly across the alveolar membrane, so the partial pressure in the alveolar gas is the same as the partial pressure in the bloodstream. It takes only about a third of the total blood flow through the pulmonary capillaries for the oxygen to equilibrate. This means that oxygen gas flow is perfusion-limited in the healthy person.

Exercise is one factor that affects blood flow and is a determinant in the equilibration of the partial pressures of oxygen. The vigorously exercising person has three times the blood flow than they do at rest. This means that the partial pressures barely equilibrate when the blood gets to the end of the pulmonary capillaries and the equilibration becomes almost diffusion-limited—but not quite. Due to luck or good evolution, blood flow is just adequate, and the diffusion is just fast enough, so you do not become hypoxic during strenuous exercise.

The problem with oxygen arises when the alveolar membrane become scarred or thickened. This reduces the flow of gas across the membrane so that the partial pressures cannot equilibrate fast enough to get into the pulmonary blood during exercise or even at rest. The flow of oxygen then becomes diffusion-limited so that the patient can become hypoxic.

The partial pressure differences can greatly influence how much oxygen diffuses across the membrane. If the partial pressure of oxygen is low, such as at a high altitude, the difference between the atmospheric/alveolar oxygen pressures and the blood oxygen partial pressure is decreased. This means that not as much oxygen diffuses across the membrane and you can become hypoxic, especially when you are exercising.

Carbon dioxide is different. It diffuses extremely fast across the membrane from the blood to the alveolar air space. Since it diffuses fast, it is considered perfusion-limited. There are a few diseases that affect the flow of CO2 across the membrane. It requires a normal blood flow and a normal respiratory rate to affect the amount of carbon dioxide in the bloodstream.

Oxygen Transport

Oxygen does dissolve in blood but not as much as you would think. A full 97 percent of oxygen is transported on hemoglobin in the red blood cells. This is an important relationship between the oxygen and hemoglobin and not just the dissolved oxygen. Oxygen can attach to hemoglobin when needed, and it can detach from hemoglobin when not needed. The determining factor as to whether it attaches or detaches is the partial pressure of oxygen in the surrounding area.

There is an oxygen-hemoglobin dissociation curve you need to know about. It is an important concept that helps you decide whether oxygen is going to attach to, or detach from, hemoglobin. **Figure 4 shows a simple curve and the attachment of oxygen, which depends on the partial pressure**:

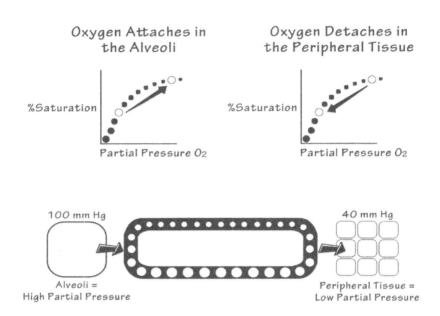

Notice that this curve is nonlinear and is sigmoidal. There is a low plateau on one side and a high plateau on the other side. This happens because of the unique properties of hemoglobin and the cooperative binding of oxygen as the four total molecules of oxygen bind to one hemoglobin molecule.

The partial pressure of oxygen in a healthy pulmonary capillary is 100 mm Hg, which is high enough for the attachment of oxygen to hemoglobin. This leads to 97 percent oxygen saturation. In peripheral tissues, the partial pressure is just 40 mm Hg because it is being used up by the tissues. This leads to the off-loading of oxygen from the hemoglobin, where the percent saturation is just 60 percent.

If the cells in the peripheral tissue are metabolically active, the partial pressure can drop to 20 mm Hg, so even more oxygen gets off-loaded. No worries though, because it will be replaced in the lungs with the very next pass through the pulmonary vasculature. You need to have enough hemoglobin to do this, however. If a person is anemic, they might not have enough oxygen available for peripheral tissue consumption.

Because of the high plateau on the right-hand side of the curve, high altitude and low oxygen partial pressures on the high end do not affect the percent saturation until the partial pressure drops to about 80 mm Hg. Drops in oxygen less than this will result in far less oxygen attaching to hemoglobin. This might happen at extremely high altitudes. In addition, because of this plateau, giving oxygen to a healthy person does not really do much to increase the percent saturation. **Figure 5 illustrates what this looks like:**

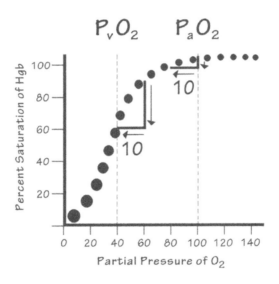

Now that you understand this curve, you need to know that there are things that can shift the curve to the left and things that can shift the curve to the right. Shifting to the left onloads more oxygen, while shifting to the right causes more oxygen to offload. Things you need to know about to understand how this works include temperature, carbon dioxide tension, and pH.

Metabolically active tissues are hotter, have higher carbon dioxide tensions, and lower pH levels. They also really, really need oxygen, so the curve shifts toward off-loading more oxygen. Each of these factors (high temperature, high CO2 levels, and low pH) shift the curve to the right so there is a decreased affinity of hemoglobin for oxygen. Fetal hemoglobin and carbon monoxide shift the curve to the left. **This is seen in Figure 6:**

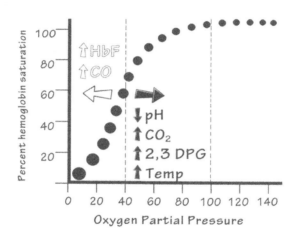

Someone has to take credit for these things, so we have the "Bohr Effect," which says that high carbon dioxide levels and decreased pH levels result in a lower hemoglobin affinity for oxygen and a right shift of the curve. More oxygen is off-loaded because the tissues really need it. The pH gets lower with CO2 because an enzyme called carbonic anhydrase in red blood cells makes carbonic acid out of CO2, releasing a hydrogen ion, which lowers the pH.

High temperatures in metabolically active tissues make for a rightward shift and a decreased affinity of hemoglobin for oxygen. This temperature increase allows for more oxygen to get to hot, active tissues, such as skeletal muscle. Again, the cells that need oxygen the most can get it.

One more thing you get out of metabolically active tissue is an intermediate molecule called 2,3-diphosphogycerate. It comes out of glycolysis in the red blood cells. If there is tissue hypoxia, the level of 2,3 DPG goes way up. This shifts the curve to the right so that more oxygen can quickly get off-loaded where it is most needed.

Hemoglobin F, or fetal hemoglobin, has a higher affinity for oxygen. It really needs this if the fetus is going to steal oxygen from the mother's circulation. Fetal hemoglobin has twenty times the affinity of oxygen compared to adult hemoglobin. This allows the fetus to be well oxygenated.

Hemoglobin will attach to carbon monoxide to a greater degree than oxygen; it is over a hundred times more attachable. While inhaling carbon monoxide is generally a bad thing for people, the body has a way of counteracting this somewhat by shifting the hemoglobin-oxygen saturation curve to the left so that oxygen attaches better to hemoglobin. The problem is that carbon monoxide is relatively irreversibly bound to hemoglobin, so it takes things like hyperbaric oxygen therapy to rip it away from the hemoglobin molecule. In addition, a leftward shift means that oxygen will not off-load well in the tissues—another big problem with carbon monoxide.

Carbon Dioxide Transport

Carbon dioxide, as you know, is a by-product (or waste product) of metabolism. It needs to travel to the lungs and get out of the system. It gets transported in three ways: dissolved in blood, bound to hemoglobin, and chemically modified (as bicarbonate).

About 5 to 10 percent of CO_2 is dissolved in the blood plasma. It diffuses out of the venous blood and into the alveolar air space (where you breathe it out). About 70 percent of it becomes bicarbonate, which, of course, cannot diffuse out of the alveolar respiratory membrane. Red blood cells have a large amount of carbonic anhydrase that makes carbonic acid out of CO_2. This turns into a hydrogen ion plus bicarbonate.

The bicarbonate gets into the plasma (and out of the red blood cell) through a bicarbonate-chloride antiporter transport system. In the lungs, the bicarbonate gets turned back into CO_2, where it leaves the blood through diffusion. High oxygen tensions make this happen to a greater degree, which is convenient because high oxygen tensions occur in the lungs. This effect is called the Haldane effect.

About 20 percent of carbon dioxide attaches to hemoglobin in the peripheral tissues. This process makes what is called "carbaminohemoglobin." Carbon dioxide gets tugged off the hemoglobin in the lungs so it can diffuse out of the alveolar capillaries. Because of the Haldane effect, this happens faster and better in conditions of high oxygen tension in the lungs.

According to Haldane, more oxygen means less carbon dioxide attaches to hemoglobin. This is the mirror image of the Bohr Effect. Oxygen and hemoglobin are competitive with one another. Oxygen is tacked on when necessary and carbon dioxide gets its turn when necessary. Oxygen-hemoglobin together means hemoglobin is more acidic. This causes bicarbonate in the plasma to be pushed toward CO_2 and outward diffusion of the gas in the lungs.

Ventilation and Perfusion

It makes sense that you need both ventilation (gas diffusion) and perfusion (blood flow) to match in the lungs. If air/oxygen is available but there is no blood perfusion, nothing happens. In the same way, if you have blood flowing to alveoli that have no oxygen or air, nothing will happen. It turns out, however, that even in healthy situations, the lungs are not perfect and there is a ventilation-perfusion distribution mismatch that can occur. In cases of pneumonia with consolidation or a pulmonary embolism, this mismatch can be great enough to cause hypoxia.

Alveolar air is refreshed with each breath. Carbon dioxide leaves with each exhalation. This leads to certain partial pressures of oxygen and carbon dioxide in the alveolar space. The amount of each gas in the alveoli depends on a balance between ventilation and perfusion. In goes the oxygen and out goes the carbon dioxide—this is called alveolar ventilation. Of course, the alveoli do not squeeze out every bit of carbon dioxide during expiration, so there is some oxygen and some carbon dioxide left in these air sacs.

Increasing ventilation (breath depth and rate) will increase the amount of fresh air that gets to the alveoli and will increase the rate at which carbon dioxide exits the lungs. This whole process will change the concentrations (partial pressures) of oxygen and CO2 in the lungs, so it will also change the difference between the partial pressures of these gases in the alveoli and blood. This can change the diffusion of these gases. There is bulk flow of these gases from the terminal bronchioles and outward, but only diffusion of these gases (which is random) in the alveoli themselves.

The blood that gets to the alveoli has lots of CO2 and very little O2. This affects the diffusion of these gases through the respiratory membrane in the alveoli, which means that pulmonary perfusion to the alveoli will affect the rate of gas diffusion in the lungs.

Alveolar CO2 Levels

The partial pressure of CO_2 in the alveolar air depends on diffusion of the gas out of the pulmonary capillaries. It also depends on how fast the CO_2 can be expelled in the breathing process. These things must balance each other out to have a low enough CO_2 partial pressure to continue the outflow process. The more CO_2 is generated, such as with heavy exercise, the faster and deeper you breathe so CO_2 can be expelled. If you hyperventilate and push more CO_2 out of the lungs, the CO_2 level will drop in the bloodstream. Your body does not like this, as you will see in a later chapter.

Because CO_2 diffuses quickly, it is the alveolar CO_2 levels that mostly determine the partial pressure of arterial CO_2. These equilibrate so quickly that the $PaCO_2$ you get from the blood gases is basically the same as the alveolar CO_2 levels. This means that the $PaCO_2$ can be used to judge the alveolar ventilation rate.

Alveolar Oxygen Levels

There are two opposing forces that determine the alveolar oxygen level. Air must contain oxygen that flows into the alveoli with each breath from the environment; oxygen must also diffuse into the capillaries which, if you remember, is a slower process compared to CO_2. The alveolar oxygen tension determines the partial pressure of oxygen in the arteries. This is because, even though it diffuses more slowly, it does eventually equilibrate at the end of pulmonary blood flow.

The partial pressure of inspired oxygen is extremely important to the alveolar partial pressure. You need oxygen from the air to be absorbed by the capillaries in the lungs for you to have oxygen. This level is about 150-160 mm Hg at sea level but is less in the alveoli because there is water vapor in the alveoli that decrease oxygen's influence. The more (and deeper) you breathe, the more oxygen you get.

The difference between O2 and CO2 here is that the partial pressure of O2 in the alveoli depends in part on the partial pressure of CO2 in the alveoli. The more you breathe out CO2, the more room there is for oxygen in the alveoli. The more CO2 you make, the less room there is for oxygen in the alveoli. In addition, the more oxygen is extracted from the tissues, the lower the venous O2 level becomes. This increases the difference across the alveolar membrane so there is greater oxygen diffusion.

Ventilation-Perfusion Ratio

As you can imagine, it takes both adequate perfusion and adequate ventilation (in the same places and at the same time) to have normal gas exchange of both oxygen and carbon dioxide. This leads to the idea of a V/Q ratio, or ventilation-perfusion ratio. It can be graphed out as the partial pressure of alveolar carbon dioxide versus the partial pressure of alveolar oxygen. **Figure 7 shows this plot:**

V/Q Ratio Plot

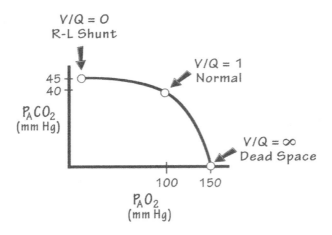

To the right of the graph, ventilation is greater than perfusion, while to the left of the graph, perfusion is greater than ventilation. At the far right, there is ventilation but no perfusion happening, and at the far left, there is perfusion but no ventilation happening. At a ratio of one, there is adequate ventilation and adequate perfusion so that gas gets completely exchanged in the alveoli. Normal venous blood has a partial pressure of oxygen that is 40 mm Hg, while it has a partial pressure of carbon dioxide that is 45 mm Hg. Inspired air has a partial pressure of O2 of 150-160 mm Hg and a partial pressure of CO2 that is zero.

The ventilation-perfusion ratio is not uniform, even in a healthy lung. This leads to a ventilation-perfusion ratio distribution that accounts for a regional variation within the lungs. In some clinical scenarios, there are significant ventilation-perfusion defects that affect the oxygenation and perfusion of the lungs, leading to areas where the lungs are perfused but not ventilated and vice versa. In a normal lung, the ventilation-perfusion ratio is the highest in the apex of the lungs and is at the lowest at the base of the lungs. This is true even though both ventilation and perfusion increase near the bases of the lungs.

Control of Respiration

How does your body keep the pH, arterial tension, and carbon dioxide tension within such a narrow range? As you know, both the kidneys and the respiratory system contribute to these levels so that the acid-base balance in the body is kept within a very limited range. While you would think that breathing is somewhat in your control (and of course, it is), the normal day-to-day activities of breathing are largely controlled by parts of the body that respond to levels of CO_2, oxygen, and pH to ensure you are always breathing adequately.

If you try to hyperventilate or hypoventilate (under-breathe), you can easily cause derangement of the body's normal control mechanisms. These derangements will sometimes lead to unconsciousness. When this happens, your unconscious brain will take over so you can reestablish a normal feedback control circuit regarding respirations that will restore breathing to the proper level.

This is a feedback system; you need sensory input and motor output for it to function properly. In the case of breathing, there are chemoreceptors in parts of the body that respond to pH, the partial pressure of oxygen, and the partial pressure of CO2. There are also pulmonary stretch receptors, J receptors, and irritant receptors that send information regarding the lung status. These do little to establish normal respirations.

In the brainstem, there are brainstem respiratory centers that act as the integration system for all the data the body collects. It is the brainstem that sends the output signals to allow for the right depth and rate of respirations in order to drive the set points (of the CO2 level, O2 level, and pH) back to normal values. Derangements of the brainstem, as you can imagine, have a very big impact on how this system works and on how you breathe. **Figure 8 shows this feedback loop:**

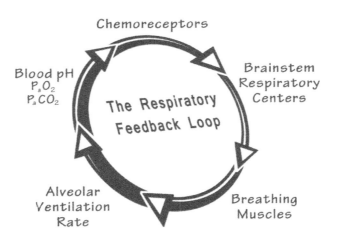

So, what are chemoreceptors? These are cells that can sense the chemistry of the fluid in the blood or extracellular fluid. Once the chemistry is "sensed," information is sent back to the brainstem respiratory centers as feedback. The brainstem respiratory centers then send out impulses to affect your respirations.

There are central chemoreceptors and peripheral chemoreceptors in the body. The central chemoreceptors are located near the medulla of the brainstem. These receptors mainly sense the arterial carbon dioxide levels (not your oxygen levels). This means they respond to cerebrospinal fluid or CSF pH levels.

Hydrogen and bicarbonate ions do not cross the blood-brain barrier, so pH changes are not quickly responded to by the brain. As you know, CO_2 can quickly cross over these membranes and can get converted to make carbonic acid, which does affect the pH of the cerebrospinal fluid. As the CO_2 level in the arteries increases, the pH of the CSF will decrease, and vice versa. This is how the pH level of the CSF gets changed by the arterial CO_2 levels.

When the CSF pH drops because of increased CO_2 levels in the bloodstream, this turns on the inspiratory centers in the brainstem, so you breathe faster in order to blow off CO_2. Nice feedback, right? The reverse happens when the CSF pH rises. It works both ways to control your respiratory rate without you having to think about it.

There are peripheral chemoreceptors located outside of the brain. The most important are those located in the carotid bodies (in the carotid arteries) and in the aortic bodies (in the aortic arch). These receptors respond to the oxygen and CO_2 levels as well as to the blood pH. Exactly how they do this is not completely clear. They appear to respond the greatest to oxygen tension changes and pH changes in the bloodstream.

Signals are sent from the peripheral chemoreceptors when the O_2 level decreases, but only when the arterial oxygen tension drops to below 80 mm Hg. This is in the steep part of the oxygen-hemoglobin dissociation curve, and this is when you most need to send the alarm that you are not getting enough oxygen.

Only the sensors in the carotid bodies have the ability to respond to changes in pH levels. These and other receptors send signals to the inspiratory center in the brainstem, so you breathe faster or slower as necessary. As you can imagine, they are triggered more by low oxygen levels than by high oxygen levels, which triggers an increased need to breathe faster and more deeply. However, you do not actually turn off your breathing when you have too much oxygen.

There are pulmonary receptors that you do not usually consciously notice. Pulmonary stretch receptors respond (of course) to stretching of the airway smooth muscle. These are more active in controlling respirations in animals than they are in humans. Irritant receptors make you cough when they are activated and can induce bronchospasm in asthmatics. J receptors are activated by an overfilling of the pulmonary capillaries as can happen with pulmonary edema. This is what leads to shortness of breath with left-sided heart failure.

The brainstem respiratory centers are spread throughout the medulla and pons of the brainstem. There is an inspiratory center in the medulla that is the main driving force behind respirations. It sends signals to the diaphragm during normal, quiet breathing. It responds to chemoreceptors and lung receptors (like the stretch receptors and irritant receptors).

There is also the pneumotaxic center in the pons. It inhibits the signal brought forth by the inspiratory center, resulting in shallower and more frequent breaths. An expiratory center in the medulla activates the abdominal rectus muscles and other expiratory muscles which are triggered by intense stimulation of the brain's inspiratory center. This allows for active expiration when you need it.

Each of the chemoreceptors (central and peripheral) and the pulmonary receptors help to modify both the oxygenation of the body and the acid-base balance of the body. Acidosis will increase the respiratory drive, so you blow off carbon dioxide, while alkalosis decreases the respiratory drive, so you hold onto carbon dioxide. These things affect the pH of the blood and CSF so you can maintain a basically normal pH level in your body.

The peripheral chemoreceptors act more quickly in response

to pH changes because it takes a little while for CO2 level changes to affect the cerebrospinal fluid pH levels. However, both will modify the inspiratory brainstem respiration center output in order to coordinate your breath rate to modulate pH levels in the body.

CHAPTER QUESTIONS

1. What does Dalton's law relate to?

   a. The relationship between temperature and gas pressure
   b. The relationship between volume and gas pressure
   c. The additive nature of partial pressures
   d. The pressure of oxygen at various altitudes

Answer: **c.** Dalton's law relates specifically to the additive nature of partial pressures in a mixture of gases.

2. What is the total air pressure in millimeters of mercury in the atmosphere at sea level?

   a. 620 mm Hg
   b. 760 mm Hg
   c. 830 mm Hg
   d. 940 mm Hg

Answer: **b.** The total air pressure of the atmosphere in millimeters of mercury is 760 mm Hg. This air pressure will decrease with increased elevation.

3. Which gas is in the greatest concentration in the earth's atmosphere?

    a. Nitrogen
    b. Oxygen
    c. Carbon dioxide
    d. Water vapor

Answer: **a.** Nitrogen is present in the atmospheric air at 78 percent, making it the most prevalent gas in atmospheric air, although each of these gases is present in the air we breathe.

4. Which gas law relates specifically to the concentration of gases in liquids and gases?

    a. Fick's law
    b. Haldane effect
    c. Dalton's law
    d. Henry's law

Answer: **d.** Henry's law specifically identifies the concentration of a gas based on a constant and the partial pressure of the gas in surrounding air.

5. What is the most prevalent way that carbon dioxide is transported in the bloodstream?

    a. Dissolved in plasma
    b. As bicarbonate
    c. Attached to hemoglobin
    d. Attached to albumin

Answer: **b.** About 70 percent of the carbon dioxide in the bloodstream is transported as bicarbonate ion. Lesser percentages are found dissolved in plasma or attached to hemoglobin.

6. What do the central chemoreceptors respond to?

    a. Partial pressure of oxygen in the bloodstream
    b. Cerebrospinal pH levels
    c. Cerebrospinal partial pressure of carbon dioxide
    d. Bicarbonate level in the bloodstream

Answer: **b.** The blood-brain barrier prevents a lot of things from passing through it, but it can respond to changes in the cerebrospinal pH and affect the inspiratory centers in the brain.

7. Where are the respiratory centers in the body located?

    a. Cerebrum

    b. Hypothalamus

    c. Diaphragm

    d. Brainstem

Answer: **d.** The brainstem has several areas known as "respiratory centers" that control respirations based on central and peripheral chemoreceptors.

8. Which feature in the bloodstream will shift the oxygen-hemoglobin dissociation curve to the left?

    a. Decreased pH

    b. Increased carbon monoxide

    c. Increased temperature

    d. Increased partial pressure of carbon dioxide

Answer: **b.** Increased carbon monoxide levels will result in a shift of the oxygen-hemoglobin dissociation curve to the left. The other choices will result in a shift to the right.

9. What is true of ventilation and perfusion as they relate to the bases of the lungs?

    a. They both increase in the bases of the lungs

    b. Perfusion increases but ventilation decreases in the bases of the lungs

    c. Perfusion decreases but ventilation increases in the bases of the lungs

    d. They both decrease in the bases of the lungs

Answer: **a.** Both ventilation and perfusion increase in the bases of the lungs, but since perfusion increases to a greater degree, the ventilation-perfusion ratio decreases in the lung bases.

10. Where is carbonic anhydrase located in the body?

    a. In the peripheral tissues

    b. In the lungs

    c. In blood plasma

    d. In the erythrocytes

Answer: **d.** There is carbonic anhydrase in the erythrocytes that make carbonic acid out of carbon dioxide in the body. This is what makes carbon dioxide so acidic.

Chapter Three:

PH, BUFFERS, AND THE KIDNEYS

We have talked a lot about pH, but what do you really know about it? pH is related to the hydrogen ion concentration in the bloodstream. The pH scale in science is based on water and has a range from 1 to 14, with 1 being extremely acidic and 14 being extremely basic, or alkaline. Every change of 1 unit indicates a tenfold change in the hydrogen ion concentration because it is the negative logarithm of the hydrogen ion concentration in water. A pH of 7 corresponds to a concentration of hydrogen ions of 1×10^{-7} moles per liter. A normal body hydrogen ion concentration is 4×10^{-8} moles per liter or a pH of 7.4.

Buffers in physiology and biochemistry are weak acids or weak bases that bind reversibly to free hydrogen ions so that there are not huge fluctuations of the blood pH level. Most buffers in biology are proteins, phosphate, and bicarbonate. Buffers will take on changes in pH and will exist either in acidic or basic form to keep the pH steady.

Buffers do not act in the entire range of the pH scale. Some are better buffers at a pH of 4.5, while others are better buffers at a pH of 9. As you might imagine, the pH at which buffers in human physiology work the best is close to the physiological pH of the bloodstream. The goal is to have an ongoing mixture of the acidic form of the buffer and the basic form of the buffer.

In the cells of the body, mostly acids are produced. Carbon dioxide is a major waste product of the human metabolism, which forms an acid. During periods of intense exercise, the anaerobic metabolism kicks in, which gives off lactic acid as a by-product. This will also reduce the pH of the extracellular fluid. Each of these processes has the potential to dangerously lower the blood pH level if left unchecked.

The two basic types of acids produced by the body's metabolism are "volatile acids" and "fixed acids." The body has mechanisms in place to get rid of both types of acids. The obvious volatile acid is carbon dioxide, which is gaseous. Suffice it to say, you make a great deal of this over the course of a given day. It becomes an acid by turning into carbonic acid, which dissociates into bicarbonate and a hydrogen ion. In the lungs, the reverse happens, and you breathe it off.

Fixed acids cannot be turned into a gas, so these cannot be breathed off through the lungs. This is where your kidneys are necessary. Your kidneys have mechanisms to get rid of hydrogen ions as part of normal physiology. Fixed acids include sulfuric acid (made through protein and the phospholipid metabolism) and lactic acid (through the anaerobic metabolism of glucose). Individuals with diabetic ketoacidosis give off other fixed acids, and the metabolism of drugs like aspirin provide even more acids for the body to get rid of.

As mentioned, you really need a stable pH level in order to have your enzymes work properly. They work best in pH ranges of 7.37 to 7.42. There are physiological buffers in the extracellular fluid that can quickly adjust to the potential for pH changes in the bloodstream. These are "quick fixes," but they are not permanent fixes to changes in blood pH.

The respiratory system—by changing the rate and depth of your breathing—is the next most rapid way to affect the pH levels. It works, of course, only with volatile acids (CO_2) and does not work with fixed acids. It is also not a long-term solution because it does not address the production of fixed acids. Long-term correction happens only through the kidneys but, as you will see, it really does not kick in very quickly. Therefore, you need the other systems in place.

The best physiological buffers in the extracellular fluid are the inorganic phosphate and bicarbonate buffer systems. Do not forget proteins, which also act within the cells to moderate the pH levels. Inorganic phosphate is a minor buffering system because its concentration is not very high in the extracellular fluid. It is a much more crucial component in buffering the kidneys and urine. It also buffers the renal tubules against marked changes in its pH levels.

Bicarbonate is the main buffering system in the extracellular fluid. It works best around pH 6.1, but is perfectly acceptable as a buffer in the blood's physiological pH levels. It has the added advantage of being able to leave the system by being converted into CO_2 gas for the lungs to get rid of it effectively. Remember, the entire process depends on going from carbonic acid to bicarbonate to CO_2 interchangeably. The weak acid is CO_2 gas and the weak base is HCO_3^- (or bicarbonate ion).

The lungs can only affect the bicarbonate buffer system by regulating the partial pressure of CO_2 in the alveoli and pulmonary capillaries. This works rapidly (but not as fast as the buffering system itself) whenever there is an alteration in the pH level of the bloodstream. It cannot, however, be maintained indefinitely. For example, you cannot under-breathe forever, or you will not have enough oxygen for the body's needs.

Renal Acid-Base Control

While the kidneys do not respond very quickly to changes in pH, they do have the benefit of exerting a more lasting solution to pH changes in the body, and they have the advantage of being able to get rid of fixed acids. When the pH is very low, the kidneys will resorb bicarbonate and actively excrete as many hydrogen ions as needed in order to maintain pH levels. If the pH level is high, bicarbonate ions can be excreted, and hydrogen ion secretion can be limited. Bicarbonate can be made anew or (de novo) and fixed acids can be secreted, making this an efficient system.

The kidneys have a mechanism for secreting hydrogen ions. This is coupled with the generation of new bicarbonate ions, which can doubly increase the pH in the extracellular fluid. When the pH is too high, the kidneys can excrete bicarbonate ions. They can also excrete fixed acids as they are made by the cells of the body. There is no other way to rid the body of fixed acids.

The tubules of the kidneys are responsible for hydrogen ion secretion. Hydrogen ions can be discarded by secreting just hydrogen ions, or by secreting ammonium ions ($NH4+$ ions). Each time this happens, a new bicarbonate molecule gets made and added to the extracellular fluid. This replaces bicarbonate for the bicarbonate buffer system. Hydrogen ions are also secreted during tubular bicarbonate resorption, but this is less important than distal tubular secretion and collecting duct secretion of hydrogen ions.

The secretion of ammonium ions happens in the proximal tubules of the kidneys. When this happens, a new bicarbonate molecule gets made and added to the extracellular fluid volume space. The process depends on the breakdown of glutamine in the kidneys into two molecules of ammonia and two molecules of bicarbonate.

The ammonia quickly adds a free hydrogen ion to itself in order to make an ammonium ion. There is a sodium-ammonium antiporter system that combines the movement of sodium and ammonium in order to secrete the ammonium ions. There is also the added benefit of the active transport of bicarbonate back into the bloodstream.

The urine can only get down to a pH of 4.5 before hydrogen ions back-leak into the tubular epithelium and eventually into the extracellular fluid. There are urinary buffer systems in place that prevent such a rapid decline in urinary pH levels. The two most important urinary buffers in the kidneys are the ammonia buffer system and the phosphate buffer system.

The phosphate buffer system involves inorganic phosphate, which gets filtered but minimally resorbed. It switches back and forth between HPO_4^{2-} and $H_2PO_4^-$ by taking on, or off-loading, hydrogen ions. This allows large amounts of hydrogen ions to get secreted without massively changing the urinary pH levels.

The ammonia buffer comes from the breakdown of amino acids, which release ammonia as part of their metabolism. The late distal tubule, as well as the collecting ducts, is extremely permeable to ammonia (a weak base). Ammonia readily takes on hydrogen ions that get secreted into the renal tubules to make ammonium ions. These same tubules are impermeable to ammonium ions. The ions get trapped and get secreted in the urine.

Bicarbonate is not secreted by the tubules. The rate of its excretion happens between the balance of filtration by the glomeruli and resorption by the tubules. Filtration is always held to a constant rate, so the actual regulatory process takes place in the tubules where changes in resorption can be seen.

About 85 percent of filtered bicarbonate becomes resorbed by the proximal tubules and 10 percent gets resorbed by the thick ascending loop of Henle. The remainder is resorbed in the early distal tubules of the kidneys. This is a complex process that depends on a balance between sodium-hydrogen antiporters, the formation of CO_2 gas in the tubules, and the reconversion of CO_2 back into bicarbonate. These cells are not particularly permeable to bicarbonate ions themselves, so it takes a CO_2 intermediate in order to get these across the membranes where they belong.

If the pH is low, almost all the filtered bicarbonate can be resorbed to keep the pH level up. If the pH is high (as in alkalosis), bicarbonate can be lost by the kidneys. This is also a relatively complicated system that is linked to cyclical hydrogen ion secretion.

So, basically, the kidneys have a great mechanism in order to participate in acid-base regulation in the body. The kidneys will make use of both renal bicarbonate excretion and renal acid secretion in order to aid in regulating the pH levels in the bloodstream. These two processes are highly coordinated. Low pH means that acid is secreted, and bicarbonate is resorbed. New bicarbonate ions are also produced by the kidneys. Alkalosis, or a high pH, means hydrogen ions get minimally secreted and bicarbonate gets excreted by the kidneys.

Keep these processes in mind when you learn about arterial blood gases. Just as diseases of the lungs can affect their ability to regulate gas exchange (and pH levels), there are diseases of the kidneys that can affect their ability to also participate in acid-base balance in the blood. Remember, the kidneys do not exert their effect right away, so acute abnormalities in pH levels in the bloodstream do not get taken care of by the kidneys for several hours (or even days) after the insult.

When the kidneys and lungs both participate to a maximal degree, the acid-base balance is said to be "compensated for." These organs are desperately trying to maintain a normal pH balance in the body so, when compensation happens, the pH can be relatively normal, but there will be abnormalities of the PaCO2 level and bicarbonate levels in order to perform compensation.

CHAPTER QUESTIONS

1. What is the pH a measure of?

    a. The log of the hydrogen ions in solution
    b. The negative log of hydrogen ions in solution
    c. The concentration of hydrogen ions in solution
    d. The solubility of hydrogen ions in solution

Answer: **b.** The pH of any aqueous solution is the negative log of the concentration of hydrogen ions in solution. A normal blood pH is about 7.4.

2. Which substance would make a good buffer in an aqueous solution?

    a. Any strong acid
    b. Any strong base
    c. A weak acid only
    d. A weak acid or a weak base

Answer: **d.** A weak acid or a weak base would be considered a good buffer because it can hold onto or donate hydrogen ions and buffer any attempt at changing the pH of the solution.

3. Metabolism in humans tends to do what to the pH?

    a. It will tend to decrease the pH of the bloodstream.
    b. It will tend to increase the pH of the bloodstream.
    c. It does not normally affect the blood pH levels.
    d. Metabolic process may either increase or decrease the blood pH, depending on physiological circumstances.

Answer: **a.** Metabolism in humans makes a great deal of carbon dioxide, which is a volatile acid. This means that metabolism tends to drive the pH values downward without compensatory mechanisms to keep the pH within the normal range.

4. What would be considered the main buffering system in the extracellular fluid?

    a. Phosphate
    b. Bicarbonate
    c. Ammonium
    d. Proteins

Answer: **b.** Bicarbonate is the major buffering system in the extracellular fluid in humans. The others have some buffering capacity but are not as important as the bicarbonate buffering system.

5. Which organ in the body can remove aspects of the bicarbonate buffering system to the greatest degree?

    a. Liver
    b. Kidneys
    c. Lungs
    d. Skin

Answer: **c.** Under most physiological situations, the bicarbonate buffering system of the lung can physically remove the CO_2 component (or volatile gas component) from the bloodstream of the body to the greatest degree.

6. What is the lowest urine pH possible before the system breaks down and allows a back-leak of hydrogen ions in the tubules of the kidneys?

    a. 3.5
    b. 4.5
    c. 5.5
    d. 6.5

Answer: **b.** The urine pH can effectively get down to a pH level of 4.5. Below this level, the system breaks down and there is a back-leak of hydrogen ions in the renal tubules.

7. Which molecule in the bloodstream is broken down in order to make ammonia, or ammonium ions, that can be secreted by the kidneys?

    a. Urea
    b. Any amino acid
    c. Glucose
    d. Glutamine

Answer: **d.** Glutamine is broken down in order to make two ammonia molecules that can ultimately get used by the kidneys to secrete acid in the form of ammonium or NH4+ ions.

8. If the blood pH is high, what do the kidneys do in order to compensate for this?

    a. Make new bicarbonate ions
    b. Secrete urea
    c. Excrete bicarbonate ions
    d. Give off CO2 molecules into the urine

Answer: **c.** The kidneys have the ability to excrete bicarbonate ions when the pH is high, which will effectively decrease the blood pH levels.

9. What aspect of acid-base balance in the kidneys is constant, regardless of the actual blood pH level in the bloodstream?

    a. Glomerular filtration of bicarbonate

    b. The making of de novo bicarbonate

    c. The secretion of bicarbonate ions

    d. The resorption of bicarbonate ions

Answer: **a.** The glomerular filtration of bicarbonate is a constant, so it cannot affect the pH of the bloodstream. Only the other factors can be altered in order to affect pH levels. Remember that there is no true secretion of bicarbonate ions—a balance is struck by the kidneys between the bicarbonate filtration and resorption.

10. What substance in the kidneys is extremely permeable through the renal tubular membranes?

    a. Bicarbonate

    b. Ammonium ions

    c. Ammonia

    d. Glucose

Answer: **c.** Ammonia is readily permeable through the renal tubular membranes. Under situations where acid needs to be secreted, ammonia will traverse the renal tubular membranes and will take on a hydrogen ion. Because ammonium is not very permeable, it gets trapped in the urine, allowing for acid secretion in the urine.

Chapter Four:

NORMAL ABG VALUES

Now that you understand the complexities of the arterial blood gases based on the physiology of the kidneys and lungs (as well as the chemoreceptors and respiratory centers in the brain), you should probably get a handle on what you should expect with regard to the arterial blood gases in the normal patient. Deviations from these values are important in understanding what is happening in your patient's body.

A normal PaO2 (oxygen tension) is 75 to 100 mm Hg. This is the partial pressure of oxygen in the arterial blood. A normal percent saturation of hemoglobin with oxygen (called the O2 sat) is 94-100 percent. You can get this from a pulse oximetry reading, but the blood gas measurement is far more accurate and reflects the percent of hemoglobin that is attached to oxygen.

As for the acid-base normal values, the normal pH is 7.35 to 7.45. Anything outside of this narrow range is acidosis (low pH values) or alkalosis (high pH values). The PaCO2, or partial pressure of carbon dioxide, is 35 to 45 mm Hg. If it is outside of this range, the lungs are the issue because only the lungs can handle the CO2 level in the body. The normal range for bicarbonate is 22 to 26 mEq/L. Only the kidneys can really change this value, so think of these when looking at this number. **Figure 9 depicts these normal values:**

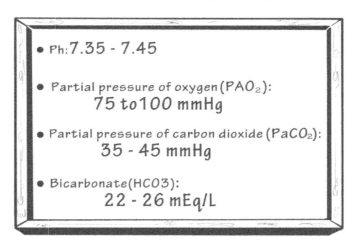

Normal Blood Gases in
Arterial Blood (ABGs)

- Ph: 7.35 - 7.45

- Partial pressure of oxygen (PAO_2):
  75 to 100 mmHg

- Partial pressure of carbon dioxide ($PaCO_2$):
  35 - 45 mmHg

- Bicarbonate ($HCO3$):
  22 - 26 mEq/L

Commit these to memory and use them in the calculations and Acid-Base problems you will see in the next chapter.

CHAPTER QUESTIONS

1. What is considered a normal partial pressure of carbon dioxide in the arterial blood?

    a. 20 mm Hg
    b. 30 mm Hg
    c. 40 mm Hg
    d. 50 mm Hg

Answer: **c.** The normal partial pressure of carbon dioxide in the arterial blood is between 35 and 45 mmHg but, when doing acid-base calculations, you should consider 40 mm Hg to be the number calculations are based on.

2. What is a normal partial pressure of oxygen in arterial blood?

    a. 50 mm Hg
    b. 90 mm Hg
    c. 120 mm Hg
    d. 200 mm Hg

Answer: **b.** The normal partial pressure of oxygen in arterial blood is between 75 and 100 mmHg, but it can be higher than this when the patient is on oxygen therapy.

3. What would a normal bicarbonate level be on an arterial blood gas analysis?

   a. 22-26
   b. 27-33
   c. 34-40
   d. 41-46

Answer: **a.** The normal bicarbonate level would be about 22 to26 mEq/L. The bicarbonate level measures the bases in the blood stream.

4. What are the units of oxygen saturation listed in on the arterial blood gas analysis?

   a. Mmol/l
   b. Mg/dL
   c. mm Hg
   d. Percent

Answer: **d.** The oxygen saturation is the percent of hemoglobin that is saturated with oxygen and so the number will be in percent.

5. What is the normal oxygen saturation level in the arterial blood gas analysis?

    a. 80-82 percent
    b. 83-87 percent
    c. 87-92 percent
    d. 94-100 percent

Answer: **d.** Hemoglobin is highly saturated with oxygen so that a normal hemoglobin saturation level is about 94 to 100 percent saturation.

Chapter Five:

SIMPLE ACID-BASE DISORDERS

Acid base disorders happen because of an imbalance in the acids and bases in the body. We actually make a lot of acid every day. In fact, it is estimated that about 15,000 millimoles of carbon dioxide are made daily—even without exercise. This CO_2 gets turned into carbonic acid. We also make a lot of organic acids, such as lactic acid (with exercise) and citric acid (through normal metabolism). The body must excrete these acids too. About 50 to 100 milliequivalents of sulfuric acid and other inorganic acids are produced when amino acids are metabolized.

The kidneys go into overtime to get rid of the inorganic and organic acids every day. Hydrogen ions get bound up with phosphate (a buffer system), urate, ammonia, and creatinine. Ammonium ions are the most abundant ion that is produced when acid needs to be excreted. Remember that ammonia comes from the metabolization of glutamine.

When the blood gases are measured, the pH and the partial pressure of CO2 (PaCO2) get measured directly, and the bicarbonate ion concentration is measured using an equation called the Henderson-Hasselbalch equation, which is complicated but accurately measures the bicarbonate level using a logarithmic calculation. Basically, it goes like this:

$$pH = 6.10 + \log([HCO3\text{-}] \div [0.03 \times PaCO2])$$

Interestingly, you can get a rough idea of the bicarbonate from the venous blood. Look at a venous blood test and you will see it does not measure the bicarbonate level; it measures the venous "total CO2" level. You should know that this is a general approximation of the bicarbonate level and is about 2 mEq/L higher than the calculated arterial bicarbonate level. It is a good estimation but does not replace the blood gas evaluation of the acid-base status of the patient.

Acid-Base Disorders

You cannot overlearn this stuff. Remember that a pH less than 7.4 (or about 7.35 or less) always equals acidemia or acidosis. In the same way, a pH greater than 7.4 (or about 7.45 or more) equals alkalemia or alkalosis. THIS IS THE FIRST THING YOU SHOULD LOOK AT. The problem can be either respiratory or metabolic (and sometimes both).

There are four different simple acid-base disorders you probably have figured out already, but we'll hammer the point home, so you really get it:

- **Metabolic Acidosis**—any disorder with a low serum bicarbonate level and a low pH level. You should remember this.
- **Metabolic Alkalosis**—any disorder with a high bicarbonate level and a high pH level. Again, this is easy to remember.
- **Respiratory Acidosis**—any disorder in which the PaCO2 is elevated and the pH is driven down below the normal range.
- **Respiratory Alkalosis**—any disorder in which the PaCO2 is low and the pH is driven up above the normal range.

The acid-base problem is considered "simple" if just one thing is wrong; the person will use either the kidneys or lungs to try to compensate for the problem. The acid-base disorder is considered a "mixed acid-base disorder" when the numbers do not add up as expected and there is trouble with both the kidneys and the lungs. It takes some clinical sleuthing to figure out what these mixed disorders are all about.

When you look at the Henderson-Hasselbalch equation, you can see that the pH depends on both the bicarbonate level and the partial pressure of carbon dioxide. There will always be some kind of attempt by a compensatory mechanism no matter what the acid-base problem is because the pH must be kept to as near a normal level as possible. These compensatory mechanisms do not always happen immediately, but the process is always underway to try to do this.

For example, when there is metabolic acidosis (low bicarbonate levels), the CO2 level will always fall in the SAME DIRECTION in order to compensate. In the same way, when there is metabolic alkalosis (high bicarbonate levels), the CO2 level will rise in the SAME DIRECTION in order to compensate. This happens within a half hour of the metabolic derangement and maximizes within 12 to 24 hours in response to the pH change.

When the problem is respiratory, the PaCO2 will rise (in respiratory acidosis) or go down (in respiratory alkalosis). In this case, there is a two-phase compensation that happens. Almost immediately, there will be a modest change in the bicarbonate level in order to compensate for the respiratory derangement. This happens because of the body's buffering capacity and takes just a few minutes. The kidneys, in order to compensate, kick in next to hold onto bicarbonate, secrete hydrogen ions, or excrete bicarbonate as necessary. The change will be IN THE SAME DIRECTION as the change in PaCO2 level. The goal is to normalize the pH level. When the kidneys fully compensate, this is called "chronic" compensation for a respiratory problem.

Let's take a look at these acid-base disorders and find out what you will see in the arterial blood gases. There are specific diseases you should consider when you see the ABG analysis.

Metabolic Acidosis

This involves a purely metabolic problem that leads to an increase in the acid or a decrease in bicarbonate in the body. While it can significantly lower the pH level, the lungs quickly compensate in order to correct the acidosis. The partial pressure of CO_2 drops, but not to the same percentage as the reduction in bicarbonate. This process of "breathing off" CO_2 is a good one, but usually not good enough to correct the pH problem, even when it fully compensates.

What causes metabolic acidosis? This condition can be due to an increase in endogenous acids, a decrease in the renal excretion of acid, or the increased loss of renal bicarbonate. Patients with chronic renal failure or renal tubular acidosis will have decreased acid secretion. Ketoacids are acids made when diabetics are uncontrolled, making diabetic ketoacidosis a common cause of metabolic acidosis. Patients in shock will have metabolic acidosis; salicylate, methanol, or ethylene glycol can be the cause of this problem. Severe diarrhea can lead to a loss of bicarbonate. Vomiting is a less common cause because, in order to trigger metabolic acidosis, more intestinal bicarbonate must be lost in comparison to the loss of gastric acid that can present with vomiting.

If it is uncompensated, the pH can be markedly below 7.35. The serum bicarbonate will be low, but the $PaCO_2$ will not have helped compensate for the low pH level. You should try to calculate the anion gap, which will be discussed in the next chapter. This will tell you if there are hidden acids in the body that are accounting for the acidosis. These "hidden acids" are not really hidden, but they contribute to an imbalance in the calculated anion gap. Things that can do this include acids that build up in diabetic ketoacidosis. Acidosis from loss of bicarbonate will have a normal anion gap because the body "trades" chloride for bicarbonate, leading to what is called "hyperchloremic" metabolic acidosis.

However, you should expect some compensation. The PaCO2 drops about 1.2 mm Hg for every 1 mEq/L decrease in the bicarbonate concentration. This happens very quickly. If the lungs do not compensate effectively and you do not see these numbers, think about either an underlying lung pathology or the presence of a neurological disease as the cause of a lack of compensation.

There are other ways to estimate what the expected arterial PaCO2 should be in a normal compensation situation. There is the Winters' Equation, which states that the PaCO2 should be 1.5 x bicarbonate level + 8 (+/- 2). Another really easy estimation is to take the bicarbonate level and add 15 to it to get the expected PaCO2. If you do not see these kinds of numbers, there has not been compensation, or you were wrong about your diagnosis in the first place.

As you can imagine, the lungs and respiratory system can only do so much to compensate for low bicarbonate levels. If the problem is extreme and the bicarbonate level is less than 6 mEq/L, the PaCO2 can drop to about 8 to 12 mm Hg—but no lower than that because, in order to do that, the respiratory muscles would have to really go into overtime and, eventually, they would become fatigued and unable sustain the effort.

Expect things like severe diarrhea to cause a normal anion gap acidosis (or "hyperchloremic metabolic acidosis") because it is a pure loss of intestinal bicarbonate levels. On the other hand, if the same patient becomes extremely hypovolemic and is not perfusing their tissues, they can develop kidney disease and lactic acidosis, which will confuse the picture and the anion gap may increase. Again, think of the whole patient and about what is likely going on regarding the underlying pathology.

Metabolic Alkalosis

This is a metabolic (non-respiratory) problem in which there is too much bicarbonate. Like metabolic acidosis, it can result in a marked increase in pH, but there are usually compensatory mechanisms that will raise the PaCO2 level in order to help normalize the blood pH value. This usually takes between thirty minutes to two hours to happen fully.

While both the bicarbonate level and the PaCO2 level will increase, the percentage increase in bicarbonate relative to the normal value will be greater than the percentage increase in the PaCO2 level. In other words, the PaCO2 to bicarbonate levels will be decreased mathematically compared to what you would see in a normal person.

Essentially, the patient compensates by hypoventilation (or under-breathing) so that CO2 can be held onto as much as possible. Less CO2 is breathed out and the PaCO2 increases, which effectively tries to normalize the blood and extracellular pH levels.

This is a very uncommon metabolic problem that can result from taking too much exogenous bicarbonate in the attempt to control a peptic ulcer. Some people take sodium bicarbonate to help reduce their stomach acid, which can lead to metabolic alkalosis. Severe vomiting will reduce the acid levels in the body because stomach acid gets lost. This can lead to alkalosis. Finally, if the patient has primary hyperaldosteronism (too much aldosterone), they will have increased renal acid secretion, which can lead to mild metabolic acidosis.

You should expect an increased PaCO2 level of about 0.7 mm Hg for every 1 mEq/L increase in the serum or arterial bicarbonate concentration. However, there is a limit to this compensation so that the PaCO2 will not be greater than 55 mm Hg, even when the pH change is maximally compensated for.

Respiratory Acidosis

This is mainly a respiratory disturbance, in which the PaCO2 is increased. While there can be a marked decrease in the blood pH level, the kidneys will eventually partially correct the pH difference. As you can imagine, the major problem is poor alveolar ventilation—severe enough to raise the CO2 level. The bicarbonate will compensate partially, but the percent change in the CO2 level will be greater than the percent change in the bicarbonate level.

The kidneys will respond nicely by secreting hydrogen ions to a greater degree, and they will decrease the urinary excretion of bicarbonate. The kidneys will also make brand-new bicarbonate ions to help raise the pH level (gradually and slowly). This process works well but will not normalize the pH level, and it will remain reduced.

What are the major causes of respiratory acidosis? There are many possible etiologies. The brainstem respiratory centers may be suppressed due to a stroke or possibly opiate ingestion. The patient's drive to breathe simply is not there. There can also be lung problems that result in hypoventilation. Severe COPD or asthma exacerbations can lead to poor oxygenation and respiratory acidosis. ARDS (acute respiratory distress syndrome), bronchitis, and interstitial lung diseases can cause under-breathing, even if the drive to breathe is there. Patients with muscular dystrophy, polio, Guillain-Barre disease, or other neuromuscular disease can become acidotic due to a CO_2 buildup. Even severely obese patients can have respiratory acidosis from restriction of the lungs.

You should normally expect a rise in bicarbonate of 1 mEq/L for every 10 mm Hg rise in $PaCO_2$ level over 40 mm Hg (which is considered normal). This response gets better over time and maximizes in three to five days, leading to a chronically compensated state. In highly compensated patients, this rise in bicarbonate can be as high as 5 mEq/L for every 10 mm Hg increase in $PaCO_2$ above the normal range.

If the $PaCO_2$ is less than 70 mm Hg, you can get a nearly normal compensatory response to the rise in CO_2 levels. The pH will still be low but can get into the low-normal range. If this is not seen, expect a "mixed" disorder with possible ongoing metabolic acidosis or acute on chronic respiratory acidosis. A pH of about 7.4 or more indicates the possibility of also having a metabolic alkalosis along with the respiratory acidosis. Always be wary of the possibility of a mixed acid-base disorder.

Respiratory Alkalosis

Respiratory alkalosis is a disease of overventilation to the point that the CO_2 level drops and there are not enough volatile acids in the system. The result is a low PaCO2 level and a gradual compensation of this low level will result in a reduction in bicarbonate in the arterial blood. Just remember, "compensation" is not the same thing as a "mixed" disorder. Compensation is understood to happen and is predictable, whereas a "mixed" pattern is unpredictable and not a normal response.

The main cause of respiratory alkalosis is hyperventilation. The lungs simply "breathe off" CO2 so the level drops dramatically. The bicarbonate level will drop as well, but the percentage change in the PaCO2 level is greater than the percentage change in the bicarbonate level. The result is alkalosis.

The kidneys will excrete more bicarbonate as a result of the alkalosis. Normally, bicarbonate is relatively conserved, but this does not happen in alkalosis. Potentially, large amounts of bicarbonate can be excreted from the kidneys. Will this be enough to bring the pH to normal? Of course not; the patient will continue to be mildly alkalotic even with the compensatory renal response.

Always think of hyperventilation as the major cause of respiratory alkalosis. Another possible cause could be a ventilator problem, in which the patient is overventilated. People at a high altitude may also breathe faster than is normal in order to try to grab as much oxygen from the high-altitude air as possible.

The expected response to respiratory alkalosis is to have a

reduction in serum bicarbonate of about 2 mEq/L for every 10 mm Hg reduction in the PaCO2 from the normal 40 mm Hg. This can increase over time to a reduction in bicarbonate of as much as 5 mEq/L for every 10 mm Hg reduction in the PaCO2 level.

Mixed Acid-Base Disorders

Any time you do not get the expected response out of the lungs from a metabolic disease, or out of the kidneys for a respiratory disease, you must entertain the possibility that you are dealing with a mixed acid-base disorder. The response can be submaximal, or it can be excessive, depending on the situation. Always look at the patient's history when determining the acid-base status. If, for example, it has not been that long since the derangement took place, the compensatory response might not be what is expected. This is not a mixed disorder but simply a lack of adequate compensation.

A mixed disorder requires a bit more analysis to decide what is occurring. The patient with salicylate intoxication, for example, is likely to have metabolic acidosis along with respiratory alkalosis. The vomiting patient can have both metabolic alkalosis and metabolic acidosis. How can this be? The vomiting will cause a reduction in stomach acid (loss of hydrogen ions) and also hypovolemic shock with lactic acidosis.

Again, look hard at the patient and think about what is happening inside their body. Vomiting usually results in metabolic alkalosis, while diarrhea usually causes metabolic acidosis. Derangements in cellular metabolism usually cause metabolic acidosis. Certain poisonings can cause metabolic acidosis. Diabetics are prone to ketoacidosis (which is a form of metabolic acidosis). The respiratory component is simpler. Either the patient is under-breathing (underventilation) or they are over-breathing (overventilation). The PaCO2 level will clearly reflect that component of the problem.

When in doubt, check the percent difference between the patient's PaCO2 level and the expected PaCO2 level. Also, check the percent difference between the patient's bicarbonate level and the expected bicarbonate level. Whichever value is the most deranged (respiratory or metabolic), that is the dominant disorder you are dealing with. Consider a normal bicarbonate to be 24 mEq/L and a normal PaCO2 to be 40 mm Hg.

Normal compensatory mechanisms will never overshoot and cause the opposite problem. The alkalotic patient will still be alkalotic when compensated for, and the acidotic patient will still be acidotic, even when compensated for. If you do not see what you expect to see, always look at the patient and look for a mixed disorder.

CHAPTER QUESTIONS

1. When conducting measurements for acid-base analysis, what values do you set for the bicarbonate level and the PaCO2 level as being normal values?

    a. Bicarbonate of 18 and a PaCO2 of 35
    b. Bicarbonate of 20 and a PaCO2 of 45
    c. Bicarbonate of 24 and a PaCO2 of 40
    d. Bicarbonate of 32 and a PaCO3 of 30

Answer: **c.** While there is a range listed for the bicarbonate level and PaCO2 level, the levels used for the calculations in acid-base analyses are a bicarbonate of 24 mEq/L and a PaCO2 of 40 mm Hg.

2. When looking at an arterial blood gas in your patient, what value should be looked at first in order to determine what the patient's main problem is?

    a. pH
    b. Bicarbonate
    c. Oxygen saturation level
    d. Partial pressure of carbon dioxide

Answer: **a.** The pH should always be looked at first, because this will tell you directly if the patient has acidosis or alkalosis. The other values are looked at next.

3. When it comes to the compensatory mechanisms in acid-base chemistry in the bloodstream, what is the goal of these compensatory mechanisms?

   a. To keep the partial pressure of oxygen within the normal range
   b. To keep the blood pH within the normal range
   c. To keep the $PaCO_2$ within the normal range
   d. To keep the bicarbonate level within the normal range

Answer: **b.** The goal in any acid-base situation is to keep the pH in the normal range. All compensatory mechanisms by the kidneys and lungs attempt to do this.

4. Poisoning with what substance is least likely to lead to metabolic acidosis?

   a. Methanol
   b. Ethylene glycol
   c. Salicylates
   d. Acetaminophen

Answer: **d.** Poisoning with each of these substances can lead to metabolic acidosis; however, acetaminophen poisoning is least likely to result in this condition.

5. When a patient has severe diarrhea, what is the most common acid-base abnormality you will see?

    a. Metabolic acidosis
    b. Metabolic alkalosis
    c. Mixed acid-base disorder
    d. Respiratory acidosis

Answer: **a.** Diarrhea leads to a loss of intestinal bicarbonate, so the patient will have metabolic acidosis as a result.

6. The patient who is predominately hyperventilating will display which of the following compensatory mechanisms?

    a. The lungs will attempt to blow off more carbon dioxide
    b. The lungs will attempt to hold onto more carbon dioxide
    c. There will be increased bicarbonate excretion by the kidneys
    d. There will be increased acid secretion by the kidneys

Answer: **c.** Because the hyperventilating patient has respiratory alkalosis, the kidneys will excrete a base in the form of bicarbonate ions to bring the pH into the normal range as much as possible.

7. What is the most common acid-base disorder seen in vomiting?

   a. Metabolic acidosis
   b. Metabolic alkalosis
   c. Respiratory acidosis
   d. Respiratory alkalosis

Answer: **b.** The most common acid-base disorder seen in vomiting is metabolic alkalosis because of the loss of gastric hydrogen ions during the vomiting process. But, under less common circumstances, intestinal bicarbonate can sometimes be lost as well.

8. The patient suffers from an opioid overdose. What acid-base disturbance do you most commonly see as being the primary problem?

   a. Metabolic acidosis
   b. Metabolic alkalosis
   c. Respiratory acidosis
   d. Respiratory alkalosis

Answer: **c.** This would be a patient that does not have the normal drive to breathe. In such a case, there will be a buildup of $CO2$ (which is a volatile acid), so the person will have respiratory acidosis.

9. What acid-base disorder would you most likely see in a patient who is not perfusing their tissues?

   a. Metabolic acidosis
   b. Metabolic alkalosis
   c. Respiratory acidosis
   d. Respiratory alkalosis

Answer: **a.** The patient who is not perfusing their tissues will have a buildup of lactic acid as part of their anaerobic metabolism. As such, they will present metabolic acidosis.

10. Which disorder results in a buildup of ketoacids in the bloodstream?
   a. Opioid overdose
   b. Salicylate poisoning
   c. Hyperventilation
   d. Diabetes mellitus

Answer: **d.** Patients with uncontrolled diabetes can develop diabetic ketoacidosis due to a buildup of ketoacids in the body. This will lead to a diagnosis of metabolic acidosis.

Chapter Six:

UNDERSTANDING ABGS
IN THE CLINICAL SENSE

After all the (possibly dull) science you have learned, which includes an understanding of the basic issues in ABG interpretation, hopefully you can better comprehend what is happening in the body when you read the ABG values of your patient. In fact, it takes the ABGs to provide the clearest explanation of not only the oxygenation status of the patient, but also the acid-base balancing that is continually going on inside the body. There are many disease states that can throw a wrench into this balance, giving an abnormal arterial blood gas analysis. Severe ABG abnormalities are not just interesting and informative, they can also be life-threatening (in some cases) if left untreated. This is what makes them so useful in the critical care setting.

When you read the ABG values, you should always be thinking of the science behind it. Are the lungs doing their job and, if not, why are they not working? What are the lungs trying to do in the regulation of acid-base imbalances? Are the kidneys doing their job, or has there not been time for these processes to kick in yet? If there has been time for the kidneys to work to regulate the acid-base balance in the body, why are they not working? Sometimes, just measuring the respiratory rate or kidney function studies along with the ABGs can give you a clue as to what is happening.

Why should you do ABGs at all if you have a pulse oximeter and a serum bicarbonate level? You need ABGs to do some of these things:

- Diagnose an acid-base disorder, which can be impossible to do without an ABG evaluation.
- Guide the treatment of a patient with an acid-base disorder.
- Help guide ventilator settings on a ventilator-dependent patient.
- Use the acid-base status in order to understand a particular electrolyte disturbance.

Getting an accurate arterial blood gas assessment depends on getting a good sample, handling the ABG sample correctly, and getting a decent ABG analysis by the analyzer. We will talk more about this later, but suffice it to say that these things are important—important enough that pre-analytic errors are a big problem when looking at a patient's arterial blood gases.

When you get the arterial blood gas value, you will get the pH, bicarbonate level, the PaCO2, the PaO2, and a base excess or deficit calculation. You should also get a relevant clinical history from the patient's lab tests, patient chart, and clinical evaluation.

If the patient has kidney failure, low blood pressure, uncontrolled diabetes, or they are on metformin (a diabetic drug), they probably have metabolic acidosis. The patient who is on a bicarbonate infusion, is receiving a high-nasogastric aspirate, is vomiting, or uses diuretics, will probably have a metabolic alkalosis. COPD patients and those with an opioid overdose, postoperative state, or muscular weakness, can have respiratory acidosis. Respiratory alkalosis is more likely to happen in hyperventilation, hepatic coma, pregnancy states, and sepsis.

Look at the ABGs and at the patient's oxygenation status. The oxygen tension in the patient depends greatly on how much air they are inspiring. The patient with a normal oxygen tension, but who is on 100 percent inspired oxygen, will probably only need that oxygen in order to bring up the oxygen level to what it would be on atmospheric air. Again, look at the patient when you are judging the arterial blood gases. The PaO_2 can be classified as mild, moderate, or severe arterial hypoxia.

In order to look at the acid-base status, first look at the pH level. If the pH is greater than about 7.4, the patient has "alkalosis"; if the pH is less than about 7.4, the patient has "acidosis." This is the first thing you need to look at regarding acid-base balance. When you make a diagnosis, it should end

84

with "acidosis" or "alkalosis"—regardless of the rest of the diagnosis (unless, of course, the pH is completely normal, and the rest of the values are normal).

The PaCO2 reflects the patient's ventilation status. If the PaCO2 is too low, the patient is probably breathing too fast, either as a primary problem or because the lungs are trying to compensate for acidosis by blowing off CO2. If the PaCO2 is too high, the patient is not breathing enough (too shallow or too slowly), so they are holding onto CO2. Again, this can be either a primary problem or compensatory for the "lung management" of alkalosis. Just a reminder—CO2 is a respiratory acid.

If the ABG is normal, the pH and the PaCO2 will move in opposite directions from each other. In addition, the bicarbonate level and the PaCO2 will move in the same direction. If the pH and the PaCO2 are both elevated or both decreased (at the same time), the person has a metabolic problem (metabolic acidosis or metabolic alkalosis). If the pH and PaCO2 move in opposite directions from each other and the PaCO2 is normal, the person has a respiratory problem.

Later, we will look at a bunch of ABGs and try to interpret them. Beware of the possibility of a mixed acid-base disorder. The bicarbonate and PaCO2 will move in the opposite direction in mixed disorders. If the PaCO2 is abnormal, the pH may be normal in a mixed acid-base disorder because both the kidneys and lungs are trying to compensate for the abnormalities that are going on inside the body. In addition, both respiratory and metabolic problems can be going on at the same time (which can get messy).

Looking at Oxygen Tension (the PaO2) in Respiratory Diseases

If the problem is a respiratory disorder (too much or too little ventilation), think about what the alveolar arterial oxygen gradient is likely to be. If there is a ventilation-perfusion mismatch or severe alveolar damage, this can lead to hypoxia and possibly an alteration in the carbon dioxide tension in the bloodstream.

Remember that the alveolar oxygen level depends partly on the CO2 level in the alveoli. The partial pressure of oxygen in the alveoli also depends on the atmospheric pressure (about 760 mm Hg at sea level) and the partial pressure of water vapor in the alveoli, which is about 47 mm Hg. **Figure 10 shows this calculation:**

Calculating the Alveolar Oxygen Tension

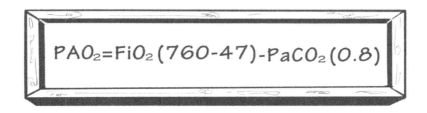

$$PAO_2 = FiO_2(760-47) - PaCO_2(0.8)$$

PAO_2 is the alveolar oxygen tension
FiO_2 is the percent of oxygen inspired
$PaCO_2$ is the carbon dioxide tension in the arteries

Respiratory failure with hypoxemia can happen with a normal gradient between the alveolar oxygen tension and the actual oxygen tension (PaO_2) in the arteries. Normal is about 10-15 mm Hg. There can also be an increased gradient between these two levels. If the number is less than 20 mm Hg, the respiratory failure is extrapulmonary (not the lung's fault).

If the gradient is large, the respiratory failure is a problem with the lungs themselves. This makes sense because, if the alveoli are not taking in oxygen, the expected PaO_2 will be high. If the alveoli are working and the patient is still hypoxic (the gradient is normal), the patient's lungs are working but something is preventing ventilation outside of the lungs.

Think about it. If the patient has a low PaO_2 level and the gradient between the alveolar O_2 and the arterial O_2 is low AND it is partially correctable with oxygen, there is a probable ventilation-perfusion mismatch. The patient probably has an airway problem (like asthma or COPD), alveolar disease, interstitial lung disease, or a pulmonary vascular disease.

If the gradient is high but it cannot be corrected with oxygen, there is a shunt happening with blood perfusing areas of the lungs that are not working properly. This can be seen in pneumonia, alveolar collapse, pulmonary edema, or a shunt in the heart or lungs.

If the alveolar oxygen content is high and there is no big gradient between the alveolar and arterial oxygen levels, the patient is hypoventilating. The respiratory drive is blocked somehow, or there is a neuromuscular disease preventing normal oxygenation. As always, there can be mixture of problems going on, so you need to think about the patient's clinical picture (more on that later).

What about situations where the lungs or kidneys are trying to compensate for a problem elsewhere in the body? The kidneys can only do so much if the $PaCO_2$ is greater than 60 mm Hg. It just cannot keep up with the respiratory acidosis going on.

The kidneys will kick in within 24 hours and there will be a chronic change in kidney function within 4 days of a respiratory problem. Again, the kidneys can only do so much. The ability to bring the pH into a normal range depends on kidney function, with the expectation that about 50 to 75 percent of the abnormal pH levels can be fixed or "compensated for" in real life situations.

In practice, the bicarbonate level will increase by 1 mEq/L for each 10 mm Hg increase in the PaCO2 above the normal level of 40 mm Hg (in acute compensation). In chronic compensation, the kidneys can do better and will increase by 3.5 mEq/L for each 10 mm Hg increase in the PaCO2 level above the normal level of 40 mm Hg.

If the patient is hyperventilating with a decreased PaCO2 level (below 40 mm Hg), the bicarbonate will decrease by 2 mEq/L for every 10 mm Hg decline below normal in the PaCO2 (in acute situations). Chronically, the kidneys can do better and will decrease by 5 mEq/L for every 10 mm Hg decline in the PaCO2 below normal.

What if the Problem is Metabolic?

If the problem is metabolic, there will be fixed acids somewhere (leading to acidosis), too much bicarbonate, or too little bicarbonate. Fortunately, the lungs can compensate to a limited degree. If the pH is low and the bicarbonate is lost AND the $PaCO_2$ is not touched at all, the patient has not compensated for this.

When the lungs do compensate, they will blow off CO_2 (acid) to try to increase the pH level. If the kidneys are not the problem either (but there are fixed acids), the bicarbonate will increase in acidosis because it will begin to hold onto it, but (because it is compensatory to acidosis) the patient will most likely still have a low pH.

What is the Anion Gap?

You can tell something about what is happening in a patient by measuring the anion gap. The anion gap is the difference between the major cations (positively-charged molecules) and the major anions (the negatively-charged molecules). For the major cations, there is sodium ($Na+$) and potassium ($K+$), and for the major anions, there is chloride ($Cl-$) and bicarbonate (HCO_3-). Adding the cations and subtracting the anions will equal the anion gap.

The normal anion gap is 4 to 12 mEq/L. There needs to be electrical neutrality, so you have weak acids (like albumin), phosphates, lactates, and sulfates to make up the difference. If the anion gap is high, there must be a lot of negatively-charged anions floating around, like ketones and lactates. This would be called "increased anion gap acidosis."

90

Remember though, that albumin counts for one of the anions so, if the albumin is low (as is seen in many critically ill patients), the anion gap may not be accurate. In addition, it is technically possible to have a low or negative anion gap. THIS IS MOST LIKELY A LABORATORY ERROR. The second most common cause of this would be a low albumin level (so look at the whole patient).

A high anion gap comes from several things. The kidneys can fail (affecting the sulfate and phosphate level). There can be ketoacids from diabetic ketoacidosis. Alcohol, starvation, and lactic acidosis from muscle metabolism can increase the anion gap. An uncommon but important cause of an increased anion gap is salicylate poisoning.

Why might the pH be high? It comes from an elevation in base (think bicarbonate) in the body. Remember that the lungs and kidneys can compensate for this by holding onto carbon dioxide (acid) and secreting lots of bicarbonate, so this tends to be compensated for. The patient who has vomited too much acid from their stomach likely has alkalosis from hydrogen ion loss. The same is true of chronic diarrhea, diuretic use, Cushing syndrome, and severe potassium depletion.

Again, the body will compensate—at least partially. The lungs can only under-breathe so much before they cannot properly oxygenate. Many of these patients can be given normal saline or potassium chloride because they help the kidneys to compensate by secreting more bicarbonate.

Rules for Quick Determination of the ABGs

1. What is the pH? Is it acidosis or alkalosis (pH above or below 7.4)?

2. If there is acidosis, what is the PaCO2 and bicarbonate level?

3. If the PaCO2 is high, you are dealing with a respiratory problem (respiratory acidosis).

4. Check the bicarbonate level for compensation (see above for this).

5. If the PaCO2 is low and the bicarbonate is low or normal, the problem is metabolic alkalosis.

6. The PaCO2 in metabolic disease is about {1.5(HCO3-) + 8} +/- 2. If it is lower than that, the patient also has respiratory alkalosis. If the PaCO2 is higher than that, the patient also has respiratory acidosis.

7. If the bicarbonate is low, check the anion gap. If this is normal, the patient likely has hyperchloremic metabolic acidosis and you should suspect diarrhea as the probable cause.

8. If the anion gap is high, then it is increased anion gap acidosis (look for other acids in the body).

9. If the pH is high (as you would see in alkalosis), look at the

bicarbonate and PaCO2 level.

10. If the PaCO2 is low, the patient has respiratory alkalosis.

11. See if the bicarbonate has compensated (see the formula for that above).

12. If the bicarbonate is high or normal and the PaCO2 is high, the patient has metabolic acidosis.

13. An expected PaCO2 would be $\{0.7(HCO3-) +21\}$ +/-2. If it is less than this, the patient also has respiratory alkalosis. If the PaCO2 is greater than this, the patient also has respiratory acidosis.

14. If the pH is normal, the patient could have a normal acid base balance or could have a mixed disorder. Check the PaCO2 and bicarbonate. If the PaCO2 is high and the bicarbonate is low, the patient has mixed respiratory and metabolic acidosis. If the PaCO2 is low and the bicarbonate is high, the patient has mixed respiratory and metabolic alkalosis.

Okay, so that seems a bit complicated, but it is a step-by-step approach to taking a hard look at the ABGs in the clinical setting.

Some Odd Things to Consider

A patient could possibly have a problem with an abnormal hemoglobin that will affect the arterial blood gas. The two abnormal hemoglobin problems to consider are carboxyhemoglobin and methemoglobin. You need to request these levels if you suspect they exist as a confounding factor in your arterial blood gas determination.

Elevated carboxyhemoglobin levels can be seen with carbon monoxide poisoning. The patient will have subtle or more obvious neurological symptoms and may have a history of smoke inhalation or exposure to the exhaust fumes from a motor vehicle.

Methemoglobinemia is usually a congenital problem, such as hemoglobin M disease, cytochrome b5 reductase deficiency or cytochrome b5 deficiency. Some drugs or toxins can lead to this problem. You should suspect methemoglobinemia whenever the pulse oximetry reading is greater than 5 percent less than the calculated percent saturation you get from the arterial blood gas. This is called a "saturation gap." The pulse oximetry can be below 90 percent, while the actual percent saturation on the ABG will be nearly normal. This is, of course, not a common problem, but you need to think about it if you do not see what numbers you expect.

CHAPTER QUESTIONS

1. Which diagnosis is least likely to lead to a diagnosis of respiratory alkalosis?

   a. Hepatic coma

   b. Opioid overdose

   c. Hyperventilation

   d. Sepsis

Answer: **b.** Each of these is a possible cause of respiratory alkalosis; however, an opioid overdose has the opposite effect on the respirations and will instead lead to respiratory acidosis.

2. Which is the major cation that contributes to the calculation of the anion gap?

   a. Sodium

   b. Potassium

   c. Chloride

   d. Albumin

Answer: **a.** Sodium is a cation because it is positively charged. It is also the cation with the greatest concentration in the blood and extracellular fluid, making it the major contributor to the anion gap on the cation side.

3. What is the most common cause of a negative anion gap?

    a. Increased bicarbonate in metabolic alkalosis

    b. High albumin levels

    c. High chloride levels

    d. Laboratory error

Answer: **d.** The most common cause of a negative anion gap is some type of laboratory error that affects one of the major components of the anion gap calculation. The second most common problem that can affect the anion gap is a low albumin level.

4. In which acid-base disorder would you need to calculate the anion gap in order to determine the cause?

    a. Metabolic acidosis

    b. Metabolic alkalosis

    c. Mixed acid-base disorder

    d. Respiratory acidosis

Answer: **a.** There are causes of normal anion gap metabolic acidosis and elevated anion gap metabolic acidosis, so it is particularly important in metabolic acidosis to determine the anion gap. It is far less important to do this in other acid-base situations.

5. If the patient is acidotic and has a low bicarbonate level, what is the most likely cause of this problem?

    a. Metabolic alkalosis
    b. Metabolic acidosis
    c. Respiratory alkalosis
    d. Respiratory acidosis

Answer: **b.** A low bicarbonate level in the setting of acidosis usually means the patient has metabolic acidosis.

6. If the patient is acidotic and has an elevated CO_2 level, what is the most likely cause of this problem?

    a. Metabolic alkalosis
    b. Metabolic acidosis
    c. Respiratory alkalosis
    d. Respiratory acidosis

Answer: **d.** The acidotic patient who has an elevated CO_2 level most likely has respiratory acidosis as their primary problem.

7. If the patient is alkalotic and has a low CO_2 level, what is the most likely cause of this problem?

    a. Metabolic alkalosis
    b. Metabolic acidosis
    c. Respiratory alkalosis
    d. Respiratory acidosis

Answer: **a.** The patient with alkalosis and a low CO_2 level is blowing off too much carbon dioxide and likely has respiratory alkalosis.

8. If the patient is alkalotic and has an elevated bicarbonate level, what is the most likely cause of the problem?

    a. Metabolic alkalosis
    b. Metabolic acidosis
    c. Respiratory alkalosis
    d. Respiratory acidosis

Answer: **a.** The patient with alkalosis who has an elevated bicarbonate level likely has metabolic alkalosis as a cause of their problem.

9. What should be considered as a probable cause of a marked increase in carboxyhemoglobin level?

    a. Smoking
    b. Respiratory acidosis
    c. Congenital problem
    d. Carbon monoxide poisoning

Answer: **d.** A mild increase in carboxyhemoglobin level can be seen in smokers, but a marked increase normally happens in carbon monoxide poisoning.

10. The patient has hyperchloremic metabolic acidosis. What disorder should you most commonly suspect in this type of patient?

    a. Diabetes mellitus

    b. Salicylate poisoning

    c. Diarrhea

    d. Poor tissue perfusion

Answer: **c.** Diarrhea will produce hyperchloremic metabolic acidosis because there will be loss of bicarbonate and an increase in chloride ions that are "traded off" to compensate for the lack of the bicarbonate anion.

Chapter Seven:

ABG COLLECTION AND SOURCES OF ERROR

The arterial blood gas analysis you receive is only as good as its collection and processing. You should know that there are many sources of error that can impact the results you receive. Getting a good blood gas is not like it is with a venous blood draw—you cannot just get a sample, put a label on it, and send it off to the laboratory. Good care of your sample is very important.

Ideally, your sample should be placed on ice and processed immediately using a glass collection tube. Gases can diffuse through a plastic syringe, which will falsely lower the PaO2 level. Leukocytes in the sample can consume what O2 is present, also falsely lowering the PaO2 level. This can be avoided by placing the sample on ice immediately after collection and by processing the sample within fifteen minutes of collection. Sometimes, using a plastic syringe is unavoidable; if this is the case, just make sure it is processed immediately.

Air bubbles are damaging to arterial blood gas collection. If an air bubble in the syringe is greater than 1 to 2 percent of the total volume of the tube, it will allow gases to diffuse into the liquid sample, altering the concentration of gases in the sample. You can avoid this by getting rid of any air bubbles as soon as you collect your sample. The problem worsens over time, so you should process the sample as soon as possible.

Do not agitate the tube, because it can disperse air bubbles within the sample. Instead, gently tap the tube to bring up any air bubbles, get rid of them at the tip of the syringe, and roll the sample gently with the palms of your hands to mix it with the anticoagulant. Do not shake it, as this will further agitate the sample.

Remember that arterial blood gases estimate the acid-base sample in the total system, but they may not be a good estimation of the acid-base balance or oxygenation you would see in the peripheral tissues when the patient is in shock. This means, for example, that if you get a sample from a pulmonary artery catheter in a patient receiving CPR, you will have a real-time evaluation of the tissue pH and $PaCO_2$ level, versus just getting a femoral ABG analysis.

This means you should get a sample from the pulmonary artery when it is possible, but only if a catheter is already in place. (It would be highly impractical to attempt to place one in a code situation.) The pulmonary artery catheter is a better measure of what is happening in the tissues of the patient.

If the patient has an arterial line in place, you need to flush it out before getting your sample or it will be inaccurate. You will also need to make sure the patient has a stable respiratory status when you get your sample. Going through all this trouble to get a sample on an unstable patient will give you a snapshot of what is happening, but it might not really aid you in your diagnosis and management of the patient.

The sample needs to be well-mixed with the anticoagulant or clots will form that will alter the reading and interpretation of the sample. Regardless of whether a small amount of liquid heparin is the tube, or a dry "bead" of heparin is present, you need to mix the sample. Again, do not shake the tube; place the syringe between the palms of your hand and roll it back and forth. Problems will arise if too much, or too little, anticoagulant has been added.

Time is of the essence with ABG analyses. If you can analyze the sample immediately, you do not need to cool it down. If there is leukocytosis or thrombocytosis, they will use up the available oxygen in the sample to a greater degree. This is another reason that the PaO2 can be artificially low if the sample is not processed within five minutes of collection. Put the sample on an ice slurry and use a glass tube if there is a significant (greater than thirty-minute) delay in processing the sample.

There are many different anticoagulants that can be used in

ABG syringes and analyzer tubing. These include liquid or solid unbalanced heparin, dry electrolyte-balanced heparin (which contains potassium, sodium, and calcium), and dry calcium-balanced heparin. Things like EDTA and citrate are acidic and will artificially lower the pH value.

Heparin is the usual additive that is placed in the sample as a form of anticoagulant. This is also a slightly acidic substance that can falsely lower the pH value. It will also decrease the $PaCO_2$ level by diluting it. You can avoid this by getting at least 2 cc of blood each time and by using a minimum amount of heparin. Put in liquid heparin and coat the tube, but squirt it back out. Better yet, use an ABG syringe that does not have liquid heparin in it.

It takes just 0.05 cc of liquid heparin per 1 cc of blood in order to have it be adequately anticoagulated. This is a really small amount, so the syringe just needs to be coated with liquid heparin. There is a 0.2 cc dead space inside a 5-cc syringe that has a one inch 22-gauge needle attached to it. This is plenty of heparin within the dead space to anticoagulate your sample, even if you put 4 cc of blood inside the tube. The diluting effect of heparin depends on the patient's hematocrit.

Always draw the recommended amount of blood per syringe when you get your sample, because getting too much or too little can make a difference in how well or how poorly it is anticoagulated. Syringes for ABG analysis will contain different amounts of heparin (dry or liquid) per syringe, so you should get the amount that will be sufficiently anticoagulated by the amount of heparin in the tube.

Heparin binds selectively to the positively charged ions (cations) in the sample, such as calcium, sodium, and potassium. If electrolytes are measured in an unbalanced heparin-containing sample, these electrolytes will be falsely low and inaccurate. Calcium is particularly affected, so consider using a calcium-balanced heparin-containing ABG syringe if you are going to try to get a calcium level off the same ABG sample.

Step by Step ABG Drawing

First, you should know that getting an arterial sample can be very challenging. This is a very painful test in the conscious patient, so when you are practicing sample retrieval and are nervous about doing so, you should draw the sample on an unconscious patient. Generally, this type of patient will not squirm and you can take your time.

What equipment will you need to do the blood draw? Use sterile or non-sterile gloves and have these things as part of your kit:

- Povidone-iodine (betadine) or chlorhexidine antiseptic on a swab or piece of sterile gauze.
- Pre-heparinized 3-cc ABG syringe with a 22-gauge, or smaller, needle attached (you may also use a standard

ABG kit, which is really handy).

- Several pieces of 2-inch by 2-inch sterile gauze, with the packages already opened before you get started.
- Adhesive wrap that can wrap the extremity after you have held pressure to the artery for a minimum of five minutes.
- Sharps container for your needles and anything else that might need to be gotten rid of.
- Plastic bag, with ice in a slurry if you will not be processing the test right away.
- Lidocaine (1-2 percent) without anesthesia. Talk to the provider to see if they would allow lidocaine can be used. In addition, the conscious patient might really need this.

A regular ABG kit can be quite handy to have. These will include pre-heparinized plastic syringes with the syringe plunger already pulled back to the 2 cc mark. There will be a needle, syringe cap, ice bag, and a protective needle sleeve included. If there is liquid heparin in it, you should expel it before using it and reposition the plunger to the 2 cc mark.

You might need to take your time getting a sample every time you get an ABG, even if you have done it several times. The sampling depends on feeling carefully for the patient's pulse and getting a direct hit to the artery right where you feel the pulse. If the sample is mixed with venous blood, as could happen if you go through a nearby vein, it will not be an accurate reflection of the arterial blood gas.

Obtain a minimum of 0.5 cc of blood, but aim for at least 1 cc. Again, read the directions on the packaging; if it indicates a specific amount that you need to get into the syringe for the most accurate reading, aim for that amount (if it is possible). The blood will be bright red, and the syringe will fill itself if the patient has the blood pressure to push the blood into the tube. It will fill briskly if the patient has a normal, or near-normal, blood pressure.

If the patient has an arterial line already in place, flush out the line and get the sample from the arterial port. This will be very convenient and will provide a readily obtainable source of arterial blood when you need it. It avoids the logistical problems involved in trying to get an arterial sample from a fresh stick.

The most common place to get your arterial blood sample is in the radial artery in the wrist, although you can also use the brachial artery in the inside of the elbow, or the femoral artery in the groin. To get the radial arterial sample, prepare the syringe as directed on the packaging. Prep the site on the wrist with povidone-iodine (or "betadine") and wear gloves.

Before you get your sample from the radial artery, you will need to do a modified Allen test. This involves compressing both the radial and ulnar arteries on either side of the wrist. Have the patient clench their fist first with their hand held high to drain the hand of blood. Release the ulnar artery compression and make sure the hand pinks up nicely after the release of this artery.

It may take up to ten minutes for the color to return to a nice pink color. If you do not see this within ten minutes, you have a positive test. It means that the hand requires both arteries in order to supply adequate blood to it and it cannot afford a temporary occlusion of the radial artery as might happen after the ABG is drawn.

The Allen test is performed the same way as the modified Allen test. In the Allen test, you occlude the ulnar artery and check for collateral circulation from the radial artery and then do the reverse to check to see that the patient can get adequate circulation from the ulnar artery. The reason the "whole" unmodified Allen test is not done, is because you really do not care about occluding the ulnar artery to see if the radial artery is sufficient. Why, you ask? Under most circumstance, you will not be getting blood from the ulnar artery.

If you are using lidocaine for an anticipated "long-duration arterial catheter" use just a half of a milliliter—enough to raise a skin wheal. If you use more than this, you will distort the anatomy and will have a difficult time feeling for the patient's pulse.

Start by feeling for the radial arterial pulse with the index and middle finger on your nondominant hand. In your dominant hand, you should be holding your syringe with the cap off. (Watch your surroundings in order to avoid needlesticks to yourself or others.) Once you feel you have the pulse, imagine the small artery just beneath the skin of your fingers. Separate your index and middle finger slightly so you have a place to get your sample.

The needle should be a direct up-and-down stick at a 90-degree angle to the skin. There is minimal angling of the needle as you would see with a venous blood draw. An angle of up to 30 degrees is, however, acceptable if you feel you need it. Carefully aim for an imaginary spot where you know the artery is between your index and middle finger. Be careful not to poke yourself. Once you reach the artery, the blood will fill the tube automatically if the patient has any kind of blood pressure. The blood should be bright red; in a hypoxic patient, however, it will not be as bright as you would like it to be.

Once you have obtained your sample, get your sterile gauze ready to apply pressure to the site. You cannot just get the sample and hold pressure for a few seconds like you can for venous samples. You will need to push firmly on the artery for about five minutes after getting the ABG. Ideally, you can have someone do this for you so you can further prepare the sample. Remember, it needs to be taken to the lab as soon as possible and mixed correctly prior to being processed.

If the patient is on blood thinners, you should hold pressure on the artery for about fifteen minutes (no peeking to see if the artery has clotted, or you will have an immediate hematoma at the site). After you have maintained pressure, verify that the bleeding has indeed stopped and wrap the wrist firmly with a pressure bandage. Then leave that pressure bandage on for about an hour after the sample has been taken. Do not make it so tight, however, that you cut off the patient's hand circulation during that period of time.

Babies do not need to have arterial whole blood in order to get a good sample. You can use a heel stick in order to get their arterial blood gas or you can draw a sample from the umbilical cord. The newborn who is having difficulty breathing should have both an arterial and venous cord blood sample collected and tested separately to assess the ABG.

If you are trying to get a "room air" sample and the patient is on oxygen, you should turn the oxygen off for about twenty to thirty minutes before getting your patient's arterial blood gas. If this cannot be tolerated by the patient, talk to the provider and set an oxygen level that is appropriate. Make sure you take note of how much oxygen the patient is on at the time you get the sample because this needs to be known in order to interpret the blood gas. Remember the FiO2 (or "fraction of inspired oxygen") is sometimes used to see if the arterial PaO2 in the patient is as expected given the amount of oxygen they are on.

The technical expertise required in order to get an arterial blood gas analysis on your patient is considerable, so do not panic if you do not get it right the first time. Patients who require vasopressors, have poor pulses from atherosclerosis, are in shock, or have arterial wall calcification, will be very difficult to stick. Ideally, the patient should be able to tip their wrist back for the best radial artery access, but this is not always possible if there are joint contractures. In addition, the patient who has tremors, edema, or obesity, will also be very hard to stick.

An ultrasound can be used in certain circumstances in order to get a better idea of where the vessel is located. You will need to work in conjunction with someone experienced in ultrasound technique if you are not experienced yourself. The use of ultrasound-guided arterial access techniques will increase your chances of getting into the artery and missing nearby veins and nerves. Use this technology if you have it and feel comfortable with it.

If the patient needs to have multiple arterial blood draws, talk to the provider about placing an arterial line. This takes extra knowledge and skill and, in most cases, requires informed consent. If you have used a site within the past several hours and need another needle stick, use an alternative site if possible. Make sure you do the Allen test on both wrists if you need to poke them in both radial arteries, as a test can be positive on one side of the patient's body but negative on the other side.

Other sites besides the radial artery can be used, but they require different techniques. The brachial artery is on the inner elbow (in the antecubital fossa) located medial to the patient's biceps tendon when the palm is facing up and the arm is extended. Use an arm board if the patient might move too much and insert the needle just above the crease of the elbow at about a 30-degree angle. It is a much deeper artery than the radial artery, so the pulse will be harder to feel. There is also a greater risk of hitting a vein.

The femoral artery is often accessed in a code situation because it is a bigger artery. It also does not require you to be so close to where all the rest of the action is going on during a code or other critical care situation. The leg should be extended, and the patient should be lying supine. Palpate the artery and go in at a 90-degree angle to the patient's skin, just below the patient's inguinal ligament.

The femoral artery is always located lateral to the vein in the groin. Even with this knowledge, and what you think is a good approximation of where the patient's femoral pulse is located, it is very easy to get a femoral vein sampling instead of an arterial sample. Look for the quality of the blood you get and see if the syringe fills by itself. Dark blue blood could mean the patient is in dire straits, but it could just as easily mean you have obtained a venous sample. In such a case, try again and go more laterally the next time around.

Less commonly, you can get an arterial sample from the axillary artery or the dorsalis pedis artery. The axillary artery is in the axilla and is best obtained with the patient's arm externally rotated and abducted. The dorsalis pedis artery can be felt in the midfoot, lateral to the extensor tendon of the great toe. Again, feel for the pulse and insert the needle at a 30-degree angle. This can be risky if the patient does not have good collateral circulation to the foot, so use it as a last resort.

You can do an Allen test of sorts to check the collateral circulation of the foot via the posterior tibialis artery. Elevate the leg until the skin of the leg blanches somewhat, and then occlude the dorsalis pedis artery with your thumb. Then lower the leg. If the posterior tibialis artery has enough collateral circulation to the foot, the foot will nicely pink up when you lower it to the level of the bed. If it does not do this, do not use that artery.

There is no reason to check for collateral circulation when doing an arterial catheter on the axillary or femoral artery. On the other hand, if the patient has poor peripheral pulses in their feet or evidence of poor lower extremity circulation (thin, pale skin with ischemic leg ulcers or poorly healing wounds), they probably have peripheral arterial disease and you should be cautious about taking blood from the femoral artery on the affected side.

The same holds true for the axillary and brachial arterial catheter If the patient's pulses are poor distally, they likely do not have great circulation and occluding this vessel (as would happen if the vessel transiently clots) is not a good idea.

Postprocedural Care and Complications

After getting an arterial blood gas, you should monitor the patient for active bleeding from the puncture site, poor circulation and color changes distal to the site, worsening pain in the affected area, or hematoma formation. The patient on blood thinners has the greatest risk for the development of a postprocedural hematoma. The patient who later needs thrombolytic therapy can have bleeding at a puncture site, even if it was done several hours before thrombolytics are given.

Serious complications from an arterial puncture are extremely uncommon, but you should be aware of this possibility. Things like local arterial catheter pain and distal paresthesia can happen. Local bruising is also very common, with the possibility of hematoma formation or actual puncture site bleeding.

Rarely, the patient can have a vasovagal response and will faint from the arterial catheterization. Other less common complications include arterial vasospasm, infection at the site of the arterial catheter, arterial occlusion from a hematoma at the site, thrombus or air embolism, and an anaphylactic reaction from local anesthetic. Extremely rare complications include the possibility of a nerve injury, arterial laceration, pseudoaneurysm formation, and provider or bystander needlesticks.

Look out for the possibility of compartment syndrome, which can lead to limb ischemia distal to the site. Common signs and symptoms include distal paresthesia, pain in the extremity, absent pulses distal to the site, and pallor or coldness of the extremity. These are all signs of an ischemic injury to the extremity. You can decrease the risk of this complication by rotating puncture sites during multiple evaluations and by holding firm pressure at the site for a minimum of five minutes. Again, do not peek until the five minutes are over with.

The Actual Blood Gas Analysis

If you have gotten a true arterial sample and have removed all air bubbles, rotating the syringe to mix the anticoagulant, you should have it read as soon as possible. The analyzer will use electrochemical sensors in order to directly measure the arterial pH, the $PaCO_2$, and the PaO_2.

The $PaCO_2$ test directly measures the CO_2 level by using a chemical reaction that uses up CO_2, making a hydrogen ion in the process. This is electrochemically "sensed" as a change in the pH of the sample. The PaO_2 level is measured with a redox reaction that will generate an electrical current that can be measured. The pH is indirectly measured using an electrode that is calibrated to measure the pH level. The voltage measured will be proportional to the amount of hydrogen ions in the sample. As mentioned, the bicarbonate level is a calculated value (using the Henderson-Hasselbalch equation). The arterial oxygen saturation or SaO_2 is also calculated based on the PaO_2 level.

The test run by the analyzer is temperature sensitive. The pH increases with a declining temperature, and both the PaO_2 and $PaCO_2$ will decrease with a declining temperature. Most automated blood gas analyzers are built for this and will report these values based on the patient's actual body temperature, or on a standardized temperature of 37 degrees Celsius.

In addition, some analyzers will also measure the carboxyhemoglobin level and the methemoglobin level (as this might be important in some settings). Nonsmokers will have about 3 percent of their hemoglobin as carboxyhemoglobin, but smokers can have a carboxyhemoglobin percentage of about 10 to 15 percent. Any level greater than this is abnormal, and you should know about it. A normal methemoglobin level in healthy people is about 1 percent in arterial blood samples.

CHAPTER QUESTIONS

1. What procedure is not indicated in the collection of the arterial blood gases?

   a. Vigorously shaking the sample to mix the anticoagulant
   b. Looking for bright red blood in the sample
   c. Putting the sample on ice
   d. Removing air bubbles from the sample

Answer: **a.** You should not vigorously shake the sample in order to mix the anticoagulant. This will tend to disperse air bubbles, which is not desirable in obtaining the sample.

2. Which is the ideal anticoagulant for an arterial blood gas sample?

   a. Liquid unbalanced heparin
   b. EDTA
   c. Solid unbalanced heparin
   d. Solid electrolyte-balanced heparin

Answer: **d.** Ideally, you should have as little liquid in it as possible, so liquid heparin is not as desirable as solid heparin. Additionally, it is better to have electrolyte-balanced heparin in order to have the most accurate results.

3. Which site is preferred for obtaining an arterial blood gas?

    a. Femoral artery

    b. Radial artery

    c. Brachial artery

    d. Axillary artery

Answer: **b.** While an arterial blood gas can be drawn from any of these sites, it is most convenient to have a sample taken from the radial artery.

4. At what angle compared to the skin should you take a sample from the femoral artery?

    a. 20 degrees

    b. 30 degrees

    c. 60 degrees

    d. 90 degrees

Answer: **d.** When taking a sample from the femoral artery, you need to hold the syringe at a 90-degree angle (or completely perpendicular to the skin).

5. When you perform a modified Allen test on a patient, which artery (or arteries) do you compress?

    a. Radial artery
    b. Brachial artery
    c. Ulnar artery
    d. Both the radial and ulnar artery

Answer: **a.** With the modified Allen test, you will compress the radial artery to see if there is adequate collateral circulation via the ulnar artery to the hand.

6. When you perform an Allen test on a patient, which artery or arteries do you compress?

    a. Radial artery
    b. Brachial artery
    c. Ulnar artery
    d. Both the radial and ulnar artery

Answer: **d.** With the Allen test, you alternately compress the radial and ulnar arteries to check for collateral circulation with the opposite vessel. This test is not necessary when performing an arterial blood gas because you do not care about what happens when the ulnar artery is compressed.

7. How long do you hold pressure on the radial artery after taking the arterial blood sample on a normal patient?

    a. 1 minute

    b. 5 minutes

    c. 10 minutes

    d. 20 minutes

Answer: **b.** You should try to maintain pressure on the radial artery for about five minutes after you obtain the arterial blood gas in order to stop any bleeding that may occur.

8. How long should you hold pressure on the radial artery after taking the arterial blood sample in an anticoagulated patient?

    a. 1 minute

    b. 5 minutes

    c. 15 minutes

    d. 30 minutes

Answer: **c.** About 15 minutes of pressure on the radial artery should effectively stop the bleeding in the anticoagulated patient.

9. Which arterial blood gas measurement is a calculated result based on the Henderson-Hasselbalch equation?

    a. PaO2

    b. HCO3-

    c. PaCO2

    d. pH

Answer: **b.** The bicarbonate level in the arterial blood gas analysis is not directly measured but is a calculated value based on the Henderson-Hasselbalch equation. The other values are directly measured.

10. What is the most common complication involved in drawing an arterial blood gas?

    a. Bruising

    b. Vasovagal syncope

    c. Compartment syndrome

    d. Nerve damage

Answer: **a.** While each of these can result from an arterial blood gas draw, the most common complication is bruising at the site of the puncture. This can be minimized by maintaining direct pressure to the artery for the recommended period of time after the blood draw.

Chapter Eight:

STUDY TOOLS ON THE WEB

If you still feel a bit confused and want some acid-base help from the internet, there are options for you. There is a "MedCalc" acid-base calculator you can put your ABG values in to get a computerized opinion of what is going on with the patient. It also has an anion gap calculator for patients who have metabolic acidosis. The website is located at http://www.medcalc.com/acidbase.html.

There is also a good visual guide on the web that shows you exactly how to get a radial artery arterial blood gas collection. It will not help you as much with the techniques necessary to collect ABGs from other patient sites, but it is a good start. You can find the guide at this site: https://www.medistudents.com/en/learning/osce-skills/cardiovascular/arterial-blood-gases/.

Finally, you can read a chapter called "Analysis and Monitoring of Gas Exchange," which is more extensive and talks about the entire process of gas exchange and arterial blood gases. You can find this chapter on this website:

https://thoracickey.com/analysis-and-monitoring-of-gas-exchange/.

Chapter Nine:

PRACTICE QUESTIONS / CASE STUDIES

This is the part of the guide where you get to put your skills to the test with some real-life questions and case studies. Feel free to go back to the chapter on acid-base disorders whenever you need to in order to refresh your memory as you work your way through these case studies. The more you practice looking at arterial blood gases, the better you'll get when you are caring for your own patients. Remember, most patients who have ABGs drawn are very sick, so you need to recognize not only what is normal and what is not normal, but also exactly what the different abnormal results mean.

Case Study 1: You are caring for a patient in the emergency room who does not give a past medical history but presents with a one-week history of shortness of breath. An arterial blood gas is obtained and the results are as follows: The pH is 7.31, the PaCO2 is 72 mm Hg, and the bicarbonate is 35 mEq/L. What does the blood gas show?

The patient is acidotic, so they must have a metabolic or respiratory acidosis. Both the PaCO2 and bicarbonate levels are elevated; the bicarbonate level is about 11 mEq/L above the normal range and the PaCO2 about 32 mm Hg above the normal range, indicating the patient is under-breathing. In acute respiratory acidosis, you would expect the bicarbonate to be increased by 3 mEq/L, but it is much higher than that, so it must be chronic or fully compensated respiratory acidosis.

To make things messier, you can also get the same results with a mixed acid-base disorder (with acute respiratory acidosis and metabolic alkalosis). This would have happened if the patient became alkalotic by vomiting a great deal before they developed respiratory acidosis. However, without a history of vomiting, you can assume this is chronic respiratory acidosis. You need to look for things that would affect ventilation (like opiate overdose, pneumonia, COPD, interstitial lung disease, neuromuscular disease, or asthma). The rest of the patient's physical examination and a better history can determine which of these is most likely.

Case Study 2: You are caring for a patient who presents with a two day history of diarrhea. An arterial blood gas is obtained, revealing a pH of 7.25, a PaCO2 of 24 mm Hg, and a bicarbonate of 10 mEq/L. What does the blood gas tell you in this situation?

Look at the pH first and you can see that the patient is acidotic. The choices are respiratory acidosis (which would involve a high PaCO2) or metabolic acidosis (which would involve a low bicarbonate). Because the bicarbonate level is low, the patient likely has metabolic acidosis. As you can see, the PaCO2 is also low, which is the expected compensation. The bicarbonate level should be 24 mEq/L, so it is about 14 mEq/L lower than expected. You can expect the PaCO2 to be compensated by doing the calculation (14 x 1.2) = or about 17 mm Hg below the expected value of about 40 mm Hg.

This patient has a simple compensated metabolic acidosis. Next, you should get a measurement of the anion gap, which is the sodium plus potassium minus the bicarbonate and chloride. A normal anion gap is 4 to 12 mEq/L. In this patient's case, the sodium is 142 mEq/L, the potassium is 2.4 mEq/L, and the chloride is 124 mEq/L. This is a normal anion gap metabolic acidosis. The patient has hyperchloremic metabolic acidosis from severe diarrhea. Remember, the anion gap is only really useful after you have determined that the patient has a metabolic acidosis.

One really quick way to assess the degree of compensation is to compare the numbers after the decimal point of the pH to the PaCO2. If these two numbers are roughly the same (as they are in this situation), the patient is compensating adequately for their reduction in bicarbonate.

If you do not get an expected number for the PaCO2 and it too high (as it might be if the patient also had obtundation and respiratory depression), you would have to assume that the patient also has respiratory acidosis. If the number is too low (as you might see in certain cases of septic shock or aspirin toxicity), you would have to assume the patient also has respiratory alkalosis. Again, you have the main problem isolated because the bicarbonate is much lower than expected. It is a matter then to see if the compensation from the lungs is what is expected or if it is something other than that.

Case Study 3: The patient is a 21-year-old male with a depressed mental status in the emergency department for reasons that are not completely clear. An arterial blood gas is obtained with a pH of 7.26, PaCO2 of 70 mm Hg, and a bicarbonate of 31 mEq/L. What does the arterial blood gas tell you about this patient?

The pH is low, so the patient has acidosis. It must be respiratory acidosis because the PaCO2 (a volatile acid) is too high. What is happening with the compensation? The kidneys will try to increase the bicarbonate level. In acute respiratory acidosis, the bicarbonate will increase by 1 mEq/L for every 10 mm Hg rise in PaCO2, which would be about 27 mEq/L. The patient with chronic respiratory acidosis would have triple the increase in bicarbonate, or a bicarbonate level of about 35 mEq/L. Because you're seeing something in the middle, you can assume it is somewhere between acute and chronic respiratory acidosis. The main thing you would suspect in this history is opiate overdose with suppression of respirations that has lasted about a day or two.

To make things messier, there are a couple of other possibilities that can be ruled out because of the patient's history. For example, chronic respiratory acidosis with a mixture of metabolic acidosis would lead to this if the patient had diarrhea or chronic COPD. The person could also have a superimposed metabolic alkalosis along with acute respiratory acidosis (but you do not have a diuretic history or vomiting history). Finally, the person could have acute superimposed on chronic respiratory acidosis. This would be seen in a chronic respiratory patient who develops worsened symptoms from pneumonia. This is not supported by the history.

Case Study 4: The patient is a 13-year-old-female with a depressed mental status and abdominal pain. She does not have a significant past medical history. Her ABG is drawn, showing a pH of 7.14, a PaCO2 of 15 mm Hg, and a bicarbonate of 5 mEq/L. What does the arterial blood gas tell you about this patient?

The patient has marked acidosis and a markedly low bicarbonate level. This is metabolic acidosis. Odds are good that she's breathing as rapidly and/or deeply as she can because the PaCO2 is also very low.

Next, you need to draw the electrolytes: The blood sugar is 760 mg/dL, the sodium is 138, the potassium is 6.4, and the chloride is 100. This leads to an anion gap of 29.4. This is quite elevated. Based on the history and laboratory results, the patient likely has diabetic ketoacidosis with a predominance of ketoacids leading to the increased anion gap. The expected compensation would be {1.5(5) + 8} +/- 2 or about 15.5. This is completely as expected; the patient has compensated metabolic acidosis from diabetic ketoacidosis.

Case Study 5: You are caring for a figure skater who presents with weakness and no other past medical history. An arterial blood gas is obtained showing a pH of 7.54, a PaCO2 of 45, and a bicarbonate of 38. Electrolytes are obtained showing sodium is 140, potassium is 2.8, and chloride is 95. What do the patient's laboratory studies say about her?

The patient has alkalosis and an elevated bicarbonate level. This means she has metabolic alkalosis. There is mild compensation because the PaCO2 is a little elevated. There are many causes of metabolic alkalosis including diuretic use and vomiting. Because the potassium is so low, you can suspect the patient has diuretic abuse as the cause of her metabolic alkalosis. (An anion gap calculation is not indicated because this is not a metabolic acidosis).

Case Study 6: The patient is an 80-year-old man who has a history of congestive heart failure. He says he has been sick for about a week and has been vomiting. He has been short of breath for several days. His arterial blood gas shows a pH of 7.58, a PaCO2 of 21, and a bicarbonate of 19 mEq/L. What does the patient's arterial blood gas say about him?

The patient's history alone could yield a variety of possibilities. The congestive heart failure and shortness of breath could mean he has respiratory alkalosis. Low tissue perfusion could indicate the presence of lactic acidosis. Finally, his vomiting could yield a metabolic alkalosis diagnosis.

The patient has an elevated pH, so he has alkalosis, and the PaCO2 is low, so he has a primary problem with respiratory alkalosis. Now it is time to see if there is adequate compensation. Remember, this will be your first clue as to whether or not there is a mixed disorder happening. The bicarbonate will drop by a minimum of 2 mEq/L for every 10 mm Hg reduction below 40 (if the problem is acute). This would lead to a bicarbonate of about 21 mEq/L.

In chronic respiratory alkalosis, you would get a bicarbonate of about 14 (5 mEq/L for every 10 mm Hg reduction in PaCO2). Due to the bicarbonate being higher than expected for the number of days he has been sick, he probably has some metabolic alkalosis from vomiting, with GI losses of acid. He has a mixed disorder with respiratory and metabolic alkalosis.

Case Study 7: You are caring for an older woman from a nursing home who presents with weakness. She has been taking a sleeping pill but takes no other medications. An arterial blood gas is drawn, showing a pH of 7.58, a PaCO2 of 53, and a bicarbonate of 44 mEq/L. What does the arterial blood gas reveal about her?

She has definite alkalosis and it appears to be a metabolic

alkalosis because the bicarbonate is markedly elevated. Now it is time to see if it has compensated. You should expect an increased PaCO2 level of about 0.7 mm Hg for every 1 mEq/L increase in the serum or arterial bicarbonate concentration. The bicarbonate is 20 mEq/L too high, so the rise in PaCO2 should be 0.7(20) or about 14 mm Hg too high. The value is actually about right at 53 mm Hg, so she is fully compensated.

Further evaluation shows these electrolytes: Sodium is 145, potassium is 1.9, and chloride is 86. Interestingly, the low chloride and low potassium are also something seen commonly in metabolic alkalosis.

In order to determine the cause of the metabolic acidosis, you need to check a urine chloride level to see if chloride is being held on to by the kidneys. Low urine chloride is seen with diuretics or loss of stomach acid. High urine chloride is seen in Cushing syndrome, primary hyperaldosteronism, and some diuretic therapies. Idiopathic metabolic alkalosis would also fall into this category. Further evaluation would help to determine what her actual diagnosis is.

Case Study 8: The patient is a 32-year-old female with a history of asthma. She checks into the emergency department stating she is short of breath. An arterial blood gases is obtained on room air showing a pH of 7.3, PaCO2 of 46 mm Hg, bicarbonate of 24 mEq/L, and a PaO2 of 56. What does the patient's blood gas say about her?

First, the partial pressure of oxygen is low, suggesting a

possible respiratory problem. She is acidotic with an elevated PaCO2 level. Due to the patient not having a change in her bicarbonate level, she most likely has acute respiratory acidosis without compensation.

Case Study 9: The patient is a 3-day-old infant who is not interested in feeding and has a rapid respiratory rate. An arterial blood gas is obtained on the baby, revealing a pH of 7.53, a PaO2 of 103 mm Hg, a PaCO2 of 27 mm Hg, and a bicarbonate of 24mEq/L. What does the baby's arterial blood gas say about her?

Even though the child's oxygenation status is normal, the pH is elevated and the PaCO2 is low, indicating respiratory alkalosis. This could be from several potential health problems, including a possible brain disorder leading to tachypnea. There is no compensation, so it is likely acute respiratory alkalosis from tachypnea.

Case Study 10: The infant is a newborn with tachypnea and cyanosis. An arterial blood gases is obtained on room air, showing a pH of 7.1, a PaCO2 of 40 mm Hg, and a bicarbonate of 12 mEq/L. The PaO2 is 60 mm Hg. What does the blood gas say about this infant?

First, the infant is not well-oxygenated on room air. The child has acidosis with a low bicarbonate level, which means there is a metabolic acidosis. The PaCO2 is normal, indicating that there is not compensation occurring. This is an infant who is probably not perfusing well and has a metabolic acidosis from hypoxia.

This can be best treated with oxygen therapy to enhance peripheral perfusion.

Made in the USA
Monee, IL
09 July 2024

61530445R00077